THE
30-MINUTE
MEDITERRANEAN DIET
COOKBOOK

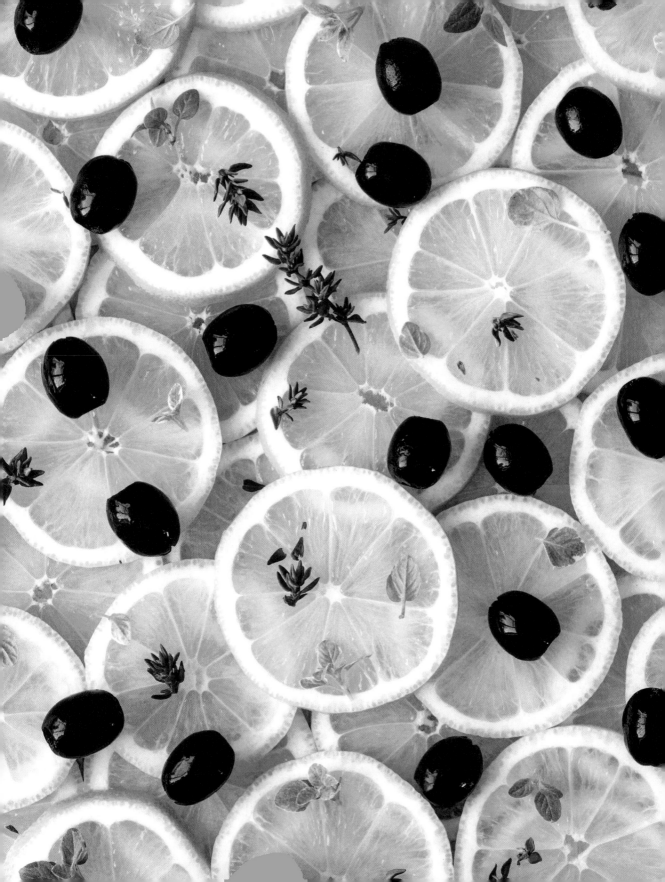

the 30-Minute
MEDITERRANEAN DIET
cookbook

101 Easy, Flavorful Recipes for Lifelong Health

SERENA BALL, MS, RDN & DEANNA SEGRAVE-DALY, RDN

ROCKRIDGE
PRESS

To Ben, who was patient; Sophia, Thea, Elijah, and Irene, who taste-tested fish recipes for breakfast; my parents, Janet and Bob, who raised me on a farm; and my sisters, who first tried my mud pies.

—*Serena*

~~~~~~~~~~~~~~~~~~~~~~~~~~~~~~~~~~

To Mia Rose; Jim S-D, who washed all those dishes; my mom, Joanne, sister, Megan, and grandmothers, Olga and Marie, who inspired and supported me in the kitchen; and my grandpop, Vincent, who gave me my Italian roots.

—*Deanna*

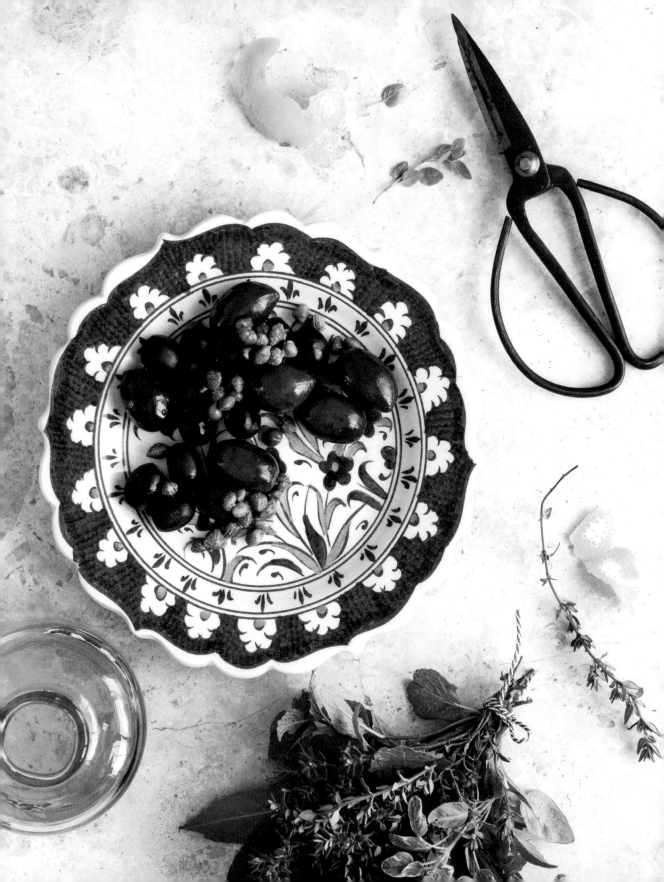

Contents

Introduction

I S there anything better than sitting down to savor a meal you've made yourself? Perhaps it's sitting down to enjoy that meal with friends or family.

Welcome to the book that will make that happen more often—in a nutritious and delicious way.

Armed with these straightforward yet enticing recipes, you'll have more chances to slow down and savor food with friends; it's the Mediterranean way, and it just happens to be healthier.

The Mediterranean Diet may bring to mind images of sunny beaches, white stucco buildings beside aqua-blue waters, and olive oil over everything. Or maybe you've been lucky enough to visit one of the countries by the Mediterranean Sea. It so happens that Serena honeymooned in Greece years ago; Deanna spent her honeymoon in Sicily and the Amalfi Coast.

Then, Serena went home to the cold, landlocked Midwest. And Deanna settled in chilly Philly. But as we've cooked for our families over the years, we've naturally leaned toward cooking the Mediterranean way, wearing both our dietitian hats and our foodie hats.

It's these uncomplicated recipes—rich in veggies, beans, whole grains, olive oil, and herbs and spices, often with fish and seafood, and at times with meat and chicken—that keep the readers of our popular blog, TeaspoonOfSpice.com, coming back.

Maybe your doctor told you to follow the Mediterranean Diet and you wondered what that meant. This cookbook will help you easily eat this way almost daily. And that's good news for everyone in your household, as researchers have shown that this way of eating day in and day out has led to better health outcomes.

We are two dietitians who love food as much as you do. And we also love culinary shortcuts. On our blog we call them Healthy Kitchen Hacks, and our readers love them. So if cooking isn't your strong point—or maybe it is, but you're juggling a lot on your plate—you'll find our hacks highlighted in the Ingredient Tips and Prep Tips that accompany most recipes in this book. They will help you prepare yummy, better-for-you recipes in just half an hour—and sometimes even less.

Here's what you'll get in this book.

- Guidelines for eating the Mediterranean way, as well as a guide for navigating your supermarket
- Delicious recipes that follow the Mediterranean Diet, and take no longer than 30 minutes to make (which means it's easier to turn eating this way into a habit)
- Better-for-you ingredients found in your local grocery store
- Recipes that focus on whole foods, not overly processed or premade items
- Mediterranean-style recipes you can enjoy even if you have an allergy or want to eat a special diet, such as Dairy-Free, Nut-Free, Gluten-Free, Egg-Free, Vegetarian, or Vegan
- Prep tips and Ingredient tips that give you even more shortcuts and insight into cooking the Mediterranean way
- Nutritional information with each recipe

Thank you for allowing us into your kitchen (virtually speaking). We know you'll grow to love eating and cooking the Mediterranean way!

— Serena and Deanna

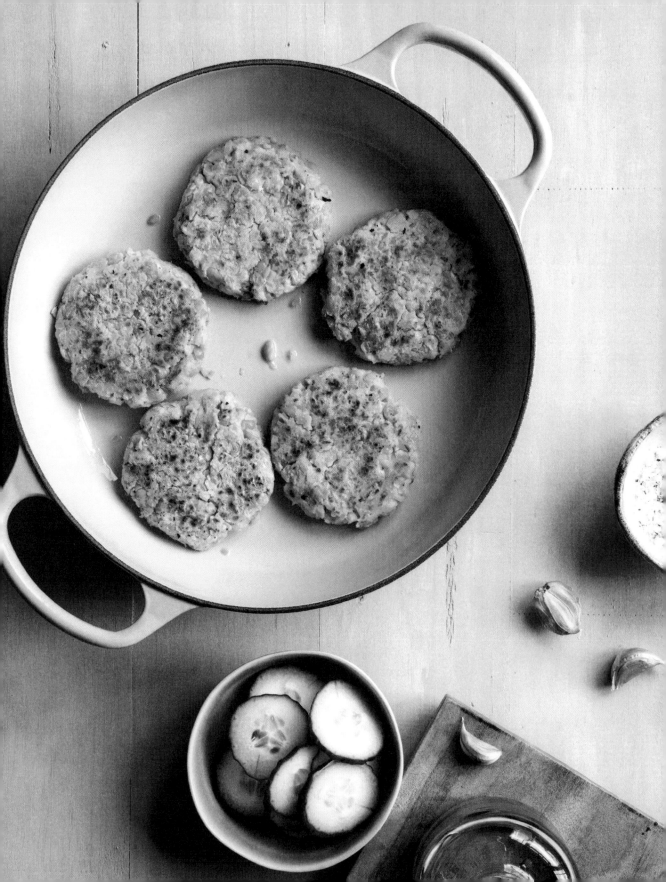

ONE

Why the Mediterranean Diet?

THE Mediterranean Diet is not some new fad diet put together by a medical "guru," celebrity trainer, or reality TV star. In fact, it's the opposite: This so-called diet is centuries older than the solid nutrition research behind it.

We don't even like to call it a diet, as that word brings to mind deprivation. Instead, we like to think of it as the Mediterranean eating *lifestyle*—an approach to eating in which you enjoy bowls of pasta and whole grains, a variety of sweet and in-season fruits, lots of crisp or roasted vegetables, slices of whole-grain crusty breads to dip into fragrant olive oil, sides of thick and creamy yogurt, abundant seafood, and aged cheeses, along with flavorful herbs and spices that season reasonable portions of chicken and meat, and a glass of wine here and there.

We hope this description gets your mouth watering and moves you out of the dieting mind-set. We want to get you excited about this new lifestyle so you can enjoy your food every day. The key to Mediterranean eating is that it's a pattern of food choices, and people in countries surrounding the Mediterranean Sea, including Italy, Spain, Turkey, Israel, Greece, Morocco, Libya, Lebanon, Algeria, Tunisia, Egypt, and southern France, have eaten this way for centuries. Each of these populations has its own unique cuisine, but what you'll find on their tables has many common threads:

- Pasta and whole grains as bases
- Lots of fruits and vegetables at every meal
- Nuts, beans, and lentils daily
- Olive oil as the main fat
- Fish and shellfish as the main protein sources
- Cheeses and plain yogurt
- Smaller portions of chicken and meat
- Fresh herbs and spices for seasoning

Health Benefits

For decades now, researchers have consistently found that people who follow the Mediterranean Diet pattern generally have less chronic disease, along with reductions in blood pressure, blood lipids, and weight. The Mediterranean Diet also helps reduce long-term blood sugar levels, according to a 2013 study published in the *American Journal of Clinical Nutrition*. All of these overwhelmingly positive results have led doctors, dietitians, diabetes educators, and many health care professionals to recommend the Mediterranean Diet to their patients year after year. In fact, it's one of only three eating patterns recommended in the current edition of *Dietary Guidelines for Americans*.

The many health benefits tied to this eating lifestyle include reduced risk of:

Alzheimer's disease: As we age, our brains shrink. In several studies, including one published in *Neurology* in 2017, researchers found that people who eat according to the Mediterranean Diet generally maintain a bigger brain size than those who don't eat this way. Some doctors speculate that having a larger brain may help lower the risk of brain diseases, including dementia and Alzheimer's.

Arthritis: In a handful of studies, researchers have found associations between eating the Mediterranean Diet and a reduction in pain caused by osteoarthritis and rheumatoid arthritis. Specific symptom-relieving foods include extra-virgin olive oil and fiber-rich whole grains, according to a 2013 study in the *Journal of Nutritional Biochemistry*.

Asthma: In both Mediterranean and non-Mediterranean countries, scientists have found the Mediterranean Diet seems to have a protective effect against asthma and wheezing in children, according to a 2017 study in *Public Health Nutrition*. In some studies, this association was also seen in the babies of mothers eating the Mediterranean Diet.

Cancer: There is a strong consensus among health care professionals that following the Mediterranean Diet is linked to reduced overall cancer rates. Cancer-lowering associations are even stronger for digestive tract cancers, as reported in a 2017 study in *Cancer Genomics and Proteomics*.

Cardiovascular disease: Most health care professionals agree that the Mediterranean Diet lowers the risk of heart disease, an association mentioned in *Dietary Guidelines for Americans*.

Diabetes: Nutrition researchers have repeatedly found associations between lower rates of type 2 diabetes and this diet. In some of the most compelling trials, published in 2018 in *Nutrition & Diabetes*, researchers compared a low-fat diet to the much higher-fat Mediterranean Diet and found that, among other health indicators, diabetes rates were lower in people eating the Mediterranean Diet.

High blood pressure: The healthy fats found in the Mediterranean Diet are probably one of the keys to the lower blood pressure rates found in people following this eating pattern. These healthier fats include the monounsaturated fats found in olive oil and some nuts and the omega-3 fats found in most fish.

High cholesterol: It's likely the Mediterranean Diet can lower the risk of heart disease partly because people eating this way have lower levels of LDL blood cholesterol. LDLs are the "bad" cholesterol, which are more apt to build up deposits in your arteries.

In January 2018, after reviewing 40 different diet plans, *U.S. News & World Report* magazine and a panel of health experts ranked the Mediterranean Diet as a Best Diet Overall (tied with the DASH diet), as well as the easiest diet plan to follow.

The Mediterranean Diet Food Pyramid

The Mediterranean Diet food pyramid was created 25 years ago by Oldways, a nonprofit food and nutrition education organization. This visual shows which foods are recommended daily and how many servings of each to eat.

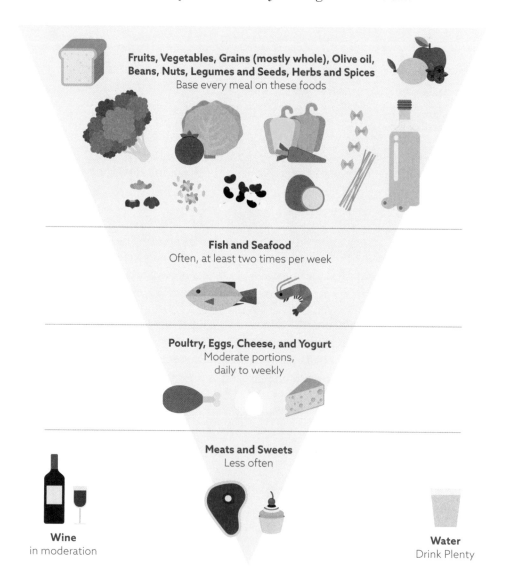

Fruits, Vegetables, Grains (mostly whole), Olive oil, Beans, Nuts, Legumes and Seeds, Herbs and Spices
Base every meal on these foods

Fish and Seafood
Often, at least two times per week

Poultry, Eggs, Cheese, and Yogurt
Moderate portions, daily to weekly

Meats and Sweets
Less often

Wine
in moderation

Water
Drink Plenty

FOODS TO FOCUS ON

Vegetables and fruits: Plant foods make up the bulk of the diet and form the largest part of the pyramid. Plants contain special components called phyto-nutrients that ward off diseases and insects. When we eat the plants, those phytonutrients can help us ward off diseases as well. Fiber-rich fruits and veg-gies can decrease the risk of chronic diseases and bulk up our meals so we feel full and satisfied.

Nuts and seeds: While nuts and seeds contain some protein, they are mainly composed of monounsaturated and polyunsaturated fats—the healthy fats that can decrease disease risk. Whole nuts and seeds also contain fiber, protein, and phytonutrients.

Beans, legumes, and whole grains: Lentils, cannellini beans, pinto beans, black beans, and chickpeas (garbanzo beans) are used often in Mediterranean meals. They are rich in protein, fiber, and energy-producing B vitamins. Eating more beans and legumes, along with whole grains, is associated with lower disease risk.

Olives and olive oil: Following the Mediterranean Diet means eating olives and/or olive oil daily. Olives are rich in heart-healthy monounsaturated fatty acids and antioxidants. Additionally, the olive fruit (yes, it's a fruit) contains healthy amounts of fiber and iron.

Herbs and spices: Along with providing powerful phytonutrients, many herbs and spices contribute to the unique flavor profiles found in Mediterranean cook-ing. Using a variety of herbs and spices will increase the nutrition, color, and fresh flavors in your meals.

Oily fish and seafood: There's a reason that seafood gets an important spot on the Mediterranean Diet pyramid: eating seafood two to three times per week reduces the risk of death from any health-related cause, according to a 2006 study in the *Journal of the American Medical Association*. It's essential during pregnancy and helps children develop a healthy brain and eyes, as outlined in a 2007 study in *The Lancet*. It's also linked to improved memory in older adults, according to a 2012 study in *Neurology*. The essential omega-3 fats in fish are found in only a few other foods. It's a myth that fish is expensive or hard to cook, and we plan to prove it to you in chapter 8 (page 95).

Poultry, eggs, cheese, and yogurt: As we get closer to the tip of the pyramid, you'll find foods that are eaten often but in smaller amounts. Poultry is eaten in smaller portions than seafood but more often than red meat. Eggs are an inexpensive complete protein source and one of the few natural sources of immune-strengthening vitamin D and brain-boosting choline. Other regular protein staples include yogurt and cheese, which contain calcium and potassium—crucial for bone health—along with probiotics, which help strengthen the immune system.

FOODS TO ENJOY IN MODERATION

At the tip of the pyramid, you'll see the words "less often" next to meats and sweets, which means they are eaten only occasionally.

Red meat: Red meat provides important nutrients, including iron, vitamin B12, and protein, but eating other protein sources such as fish, beans, or nuts often or in place of red meat can lower your risk for several diseases and premature death, according to a 2012 study in the *Archives of Internal Medicine*. So eat red meat in smaller amounts, rather like a side dish.

Sweets: Cakes, cookies, ice cream, candies, and pastries are reserved for holidays and celebrations in the Mediterranean Diet. We suggest a gradual approach in cutting back on sweets. Start with fruit for dessert twice a week while reducing portion sizes of baked goods. And don't worry; we have an entire chapter of better-for-you desserts in this book (page 163).

Wine: Wine is an integral part of the Mediterranean Diet and should be sipped slowly to enhance the taste and enjoyment of food. According to the current edition of *Dietary Guidelines for Americans*, moderate drinking is defined as two 5-ounce glasses of wine a day for men and one glass for women. These amounts appear to have the most health benefits with the least risks.

FOODS TO CUT BACK ON

Processed meats: Our big beef with processed meats like deli meats, salami, sausage, and bacon is the amount of salt and fillers in them. Cured meats like prosciutto are preferred but are eaten in small amounts and not every day.

Added sugars: We're not talking about naturally occurring sugars in fruits, vegetables, and dairy foods, but rather sugars added to a product. They are lurking everywhere these days—in condiments, yogurts, bread, and drinks—and you may not realize how much you are consuming. Look for "added sugars" on food labels. And in any recipe (not in this book), you can usually decrease the sugar by a few tablespoons. Honey is a traditional sweetener when eating the Mediterranean way, but remember, it's still considered an added sugar.

Refined grains: Refined grains are stripped of the bran and germ during milling, and as a result, the majority of available dietary fiber, iron, B vitamins, and phytonutrients are also removed. They're often found in granola bars, breads, desserts, some cereals, and sweet or savory snacks. They're listed on food labels as wheat flour, rice flour, and any flour or grain without the word "whole" in front of it (except oats, which are always a whole grain).

Sodium: The majority of the sodium in our diets doesn't come from the salt shaker, but rather, from processed foods like frozen dinners, frozen pizzas, fast food, processed meats, and condiments. Look for no-salt-added or lower-sodium labels on canned foods when buying things like tomatoes, beans, and broth. As for table salt, we use kosher or sea salt in our recipes because the granules are bigger, so you use less per recipe; but a little salt is important when cooking to make the other flavors in your recipe shine.

Empty-calorie beverages: Sports drinks, energy drinks, sweetened iced teas, and sodas add only calories and sugar to your diet. Bottom line: Drink water. (And the occasional glass of wine—and we'll give you your coffee, too!)

Eight Guiding Principles

Eating according to the Mediterranean Diet doesn't mean you can't also enjoy Asian, Mexican, Indian, Scandinavian, or American Southern dishes. You can dine around the world. Simply apply these principles of Mediterranean meal patterns to other cuisines.

1. **Look to the sea.** Seafood is king in the Mediterranean Diet. Don't think you like fish? Start with a milder fish like tilapia or cod, and grill or cook it in a flavorful tomato sauce. Canned albacore tuna tastes less fishy compared to canned light tuna; mix it with plain Greek yogurt or hummus and add fresh herbs to help buffer the fish taste for a tuna sandwich. Check out chapter 8 (page 95) for more inspiration.

2. **Rearrange your plate.** The USDA's MyPlate guide suggests we cover half of our dinner plate with vegetables and fruits. That leaves a quarter of the plate for protein—like beans, seafood, poultry, eggs, and meat—and the remaining quarter for whole grains. We practice this with many of the recipes in our main dish chapters.

3. **Savor seasonal foods.** Feeding your family according to the seasons is one of the most satisfying—and delicious—ways to eat. Eating apples and pears mainly in the fall and winter, at their peak of freshness, makes you appreciate them all the more. Biting into that sweet, juicy summer tomato or peach is incomparably better than eating those flavorless ones in the markets in winter. And nothing beats that first taste of spring asparagus. Get inspired by visiting a farmers' market or the local produce section of your supermarket. Enjoy nutritious (low-sodium) canned and frozen fruits and vegetables when the fresh versions aren't in season.

4. **Be savvy about portions.** This is one of the trickiest parts of healthy eating. We believe that no food is off-limits, if it's consumed in reasonable portions. Eating slowly and enjoying each bite is key. While 1 cup is the standard serving size for fruits and veggies, for most other foods, a 1/2-cup serving is a good place to start. If you're satisfied and mostly full (not stuffed) about 15 minutes after your meal, stop. If not, try a 1/4-cup or smaller additional serving, or fill up on more vegetables and fruit. And leftovers are a beautiful thing—a day off from cooking!

5. **Get into whole grains and beans.** Eat beans, lentils, and whole grains regularly—even at breakfast (see chapter 2 for ideas, page 17). Start dinner preparations by setting a pot of whole grains to cook on the stove, and then simply add ingredients from your refrigerator or pantry. Use canned beans as a great time-saver.

6. **Make meat a seasoning.** Use red meat as a flavoring or a complement to dishes rather than the main feature. Soups, stews, burgers, kebabs, and other entrées may stretch a half pound of red meat to four servings with the addition of whole grains, nuts, and vegetables. Four ounces or less of meat is considered a main dish serving and is usually eaten only a few times a week.

7. **Embrace herbs and spices.** A variety of herbs and spices can add flavor, flair, color, and nutrients to your recipes. Look to your garden, the produce aisle, and your spice drawer for inspiration. Experiment by adding fresh green

herbs like basil, mint, or parsley to salads or grain dishes. Sprinkle dried herbs like oregano, rosemary, or thyme over fish and pasta. Add spices like smoked paprika, cumin, or crushed red pepper to sauces and dressings.

8. **Do dessert, but differently.** "Eat dessert nightly" is definitely a rule we live by. That said, fruit is the dessert of choice in the Mediterranean Diet. But not just plain fruit—think baked apples filled with nuts and raisins, or grilled peaches topped with a drizzle of honey. A bowl of berries topped with plain yogurt and jam is often dessert at our houses. Need a dessert after lunch? A square of dark chocolate is a portable fix for sweet cravings. (For more ideas, check out chapter 12, page 163).

The Mediterranean Lifestyle

It's easy to be healthy when you live in a sunny country on the Mediterranean Sea. With the ocean breeze, sunshine, and good wine, how could you be stressed out and lack energy? Part of the Mediterranean Diet means adopting a bit of a vacation-mode attitude, at least for several minutes throughout the day. Here's how:

Slow down at mealtimes. Time the length of one of your regular family meals. Then, try stretching it out just 10 minutes longer, to include conversation with the folks at your table. And yes, please eat at a table with all TVs, phones, and electronics off. You'll be on your way to the relaxed meal that's a signature of Mediterranean regions.

Savor a glass of wine. Savoring wine with a meal helps slow down your dinners. Serve wine (it doesn't have to be an expensive bottle) on the nights you have time to appreciate it, or serve it with a leisurely lunch on the weekends. It's customary to enjoy wine only when food is also being served.

Move that body more often. You could have the healthiest diet in the world, but without moving your muscles, your body won't be truly fit. Keeping your muscles strong helps prevent injured backs and shoulders and makes it easier to do just about everything. Think of daily physical activity as insurance against aches and pains. It is also an amazing way to relieve stress. Even 10-minute spurts of activity several times throughout the day lead to better health.

Get a good night's sleep. Aim for seven to eight hours of sleep nightly. We can't stress this enough. We know people who have changed their entire lives just by regularly getting enough sleep. Even with the best diet and exercise plan in the world, your body will not work as efficiently without enough sleep. Make it a priority.

The Mediterranean Kitchen

You may already have a Mediterranean kitchen and not even know it. There's no need to buy a lot of expensive ingredients, as many Mediterranean staples, like beans, canned tomatoes, and tuna, are probably in your pantry right now.

PANTRY ESSENTIALS

Olives: If your grocery store has an olive bar (often near the deli department), sample different varieties to find your favorites. Then buy that variety in a jar, as they are usually less expensive than at the olive bar. Start tossing olives into soups, salads, sandwiches, pastas, potatoes, or almost any dish in which you'd use salt.

Beans (canned and dried): You can feed a crowd of 10 with one bag of dried beans, which costs about $1.50. Get in the habit of cooking up one batch a week. Dried lentils cook even faster. You also can't go wrong with any can of beans; drain and rinse them to remove about 40 percent of the sodium.

Nuts and seeds: Go nuts over seeds and nuts. Sprinkle a tablespoon or two over any dish to add flavor, crunch, and a dose of good fats. Almonds, pecans, peanuts, pistachios, walnuts, chia seeds, ground flaxseed, pumpkin seeds, and sesame seeds are all nutrition boosters.

Whole grains and brown rice: Whole grains are the foundation of the Mediterranean Diet. Luckily, delicious whole grains like sorghum, quinoa, spelt, and farro are now easier to find. To begin to enjoy whole grains you might be unfamiliar with, combine the new whole grain with rice.

Pasta: Pasta is a healthy, low-glycemic-index food. (The glycemic index rates how fast a carbohydrate-rich food is digested and affects your blood sugar levels.) The way dried pasta is made actually reduces its glycemic index. To get more fiber in your diet, choose whole-grain pasta more often.

Canned fish: We serve budget-friendly canned tuna or salmon a couple of times a week. (Go for the kind packed in olive oil for extra flavor.) Drain sardines or anchovies and mash into tomato sauce for extra nutrients and richness.

Canned and jarred vegetables: Canned, no-salt tomato products are a pantry necessity—especially because the tomato season is short in most parts of the world. Jarred roasted bell peppers, artichoke hearts, and capers are veggie staples you can use daily while eating the Mediterranean way.

Olive oil and vinegar: If you have these two staples on hand, you can flavor any dish (Deanna has 8 to 10 bottles in her pantry!). We like to use extra-virgin olive oil for cooking and drizzling. It has the most health benefits, and a high enough smoke point to be practical when sautéing. Balsamic vinegar and red wine vinegar are two of our favorites and are typical staples in the Mediterranean Diet.

Kosher or sea salt: You might be surprised to see salt on two dietitians' pantry lists, but remember that the majority of sodium in our diets doesn't come from table salt. That said, the larger grains of these salts means there's less in your measuring spoon, but they still deliver a big flavor punch to dishes.

GROCERY STORE GUIDE: HOW TO SHOP

Don't follow the old rule that you should only shop the perimeter of the grocery store. Today's supermarkets have Mediterranean Diet staples in every aisle—including the middle ones. While shopping, picture the Mediterranean Diet Pyramid inside your shopping cart: Half your cart should be fruits, vegetables, and plant-based foods, then fill up the rest with seafood, and so on.

Fresh produce section: What's in season? Seasonal fruits and vegetables are usually less expensive. Don't forget fresh herbs: Parsley, cilantro, basil, and mint can be budget-friendly ways to eat more always-in-season greens.

Fish counter: Ask questions. The fishmonger behind the counter is happy to steer you to inexpensive choices; he or she can also be a great source for recipes and cooking tips.

Canned fish aisle: There are lots of new additions here, including packets of tuna and salmon that are ready to eat with a fork. Most of the choices are simple and sustainable. Just pick your favorite or try something new, like sardines.

Frozen food aisle: The frozen food aisle is an ideal place to finish filling your cart with fruit and veggies. In general, frozen fruits and vegetables are just as

THE PROCESSED FOOD PUZZLE

These days, the term "processed food" is often associated with negative qualities, when in reality, a processed food is any food that has been changed in some way before consumption. This includes all frozen, canned, cooked, or fortified foods. And while there are certainly processed foods we'd recommend eating less of, there are also many staples in the Mediterranean Diet that go through some kind of processing for preservation and food safety, like dried grains, frozen produce, and canned beans.

Typically, the processed foods that are more problematic have long lists of ingredients, including many terms you might not even recognize. Many are high in sodium, saturated fat, artificial flavors, and other undesirable ingredients we want to eat less of and even avoid when possible. When in doubt about a food, check the label for the amount of added sugar, sodium, saturated fat, and extra ingredients.

To help you when shopping, here's a basic list of minimally processed foods that we recommend and a list of overly processed foods to eat less of.

Minimally processed:

- Canned fish
- Dried pasta, grains (without any additional ingredients)
- Frozen fish, vegetables, and fruits
- Plain yogurt
- Extra-virgin olive oil
- Canned beans, vegetables, and fruits
- Bagged produce

Highly processed (depending on the brand, some of these items may be less processed than others):

- Frozen dinners
- Frozen pizzas
- Fast food
- Deli meats, sausage, and bacon
- Salad dressings, condiments, and sauces
- Crackers and chips
- Shelf-stable baked goods

nutritious as fresh, as they are frozen at the peak of freshness. Choose any vegetable without sauce. We buy frozen fruits to go into every breakfast, from cereal to yogurt. Frozen fish fillets are healthy, convenient choices, and because they're often frozen individually, you can cook just what you need.

Rice and grains aisle: In general, you'll find most whole grains here, in the natural foods aisle, or in the bulk food section. To make sure the grains are whole, search for these words on the Nutrition Facts label: oats, bulgur, wheat berries, rye berries, or whole [name of grain], such as whole wheat. Look for farro, bulgur, quinoa, sorghum, spelt, barley, brown rice (instant and regular), and wild rice without any added flavors or seasonings.

Bulk food section: This area, with foods in open bins, makes food shopping fun. Here's where you can buy small amounts of things to taste, without spending a lot on full packages of whole grains, beans, and dried fruits.

Dairy case: From low-fat to full-fat, we promote eating the type of milk, cheese, or yogurt that you prefer. Products with more fat will have more calories, but we find that they are more filling and flavorful, and often you can use less in a recipe. When it comes to yogurt, we prefer plain, but if you are buying flavored yogurt, compare the amount of added sugar to other flavored yogurts and go with the lowest number. (The total sugar amount on the label also includes the lactose and fructose—those naturally occurring sugars found in dairy and fruit.) Or better yet, buy the plain and add your own fruit.

Your Basic Tools

The recipes in this book use basic kitchen equipment you probably already have. Here's a list of the kitchen tools we use most often.

- Chef's knife
- Paring knife
- Two (12-by-18-inch) half sheet pans, also known as rimmed baking sheets (in the recipes, this is what we'll call a large rimmed baking sheet)
- Large (10- or 12-inch) nonstick skillet with a lid, or cast iron skillet (in the recipes, this is what we'll call a large skillet)
- 8-quart covered stockpot for soups and stews (in the recipes, this is what we'll call a large stockpot)

- 4-quart covered saucepan or pot to cook whole grains or vegetables (in the recipes, this is what we'll call a medium saucepan)
- 9-by-13-inch baking pan for roasting vegetables (in the recipes, this is what we'll call a baking pan)
- Meat thermometer
- Ruler
- Kitchen brush
- Microplane zester for grating citrus
- Two mixing bowls: one large and one medium
- Measuring cups and spoons
- Fine mesh strainer for straining citrus juice
- Colander for draining canned beans, pasta, and grains
- Two cutting boards—one for produce and one for meat, poultry, and fish
- Glass containers for food storage and leftovers
- Blender and/or immersion blender
- Food processor

About the Recipes

Friends and family—from novices to experienced cooks—helped us test the recipes in this book. While each of these recipes takes around 30 minutes or less, keep in mind that the prep and cooking times are our best estimates. Different people (and different ovens) do things at different speeds. And we often are prepping ingredients while something is cooking in the oven or on the stove, which is reflected in the cooking times.

We always recommend that you first read the recipe all the way through and get all your ingredients out before diving in. This will ultimately save you time in the kitchen—and make sure your dinner is done in around 30 minutes or less!

If you're cooking for family or guests with varied tastes or special dietary needs, we've got you covered. Look for the following labels:

- Dairy-free
- Nut-free
- Gluten-free
- Egg-free
- Vegetarian
- Vegan
- 5 ingredients (not including water, salt, pepper, oil, and nonstick cooking spray)
- One pot (the recipe can be cooked in a single pot or pan or baking dish)
- Half the time (15 minutes or less from start to finish, including all the prep and cooking)

Remember to always check labels while you shop, though. For example, some ingredients like oats are naturally gluten-free but processed in factories with cross contamination. If gluten or nuts are a concern for you, be sure to look out for labels on packaging before you buy or use anything.

And if you remember only one thing, remember this: The Mediterranean Diet is NOT a strict diet.

It's a pattern of eating based on vegetables, fruits, whole grains, fish, beans, nuts, olive oil, and some dairy and meat. Please swap ingredients in and out of our recipes based on your preferences.

What we mean is, use brown rice if you don't have quinoa. Use spinach if you don't like kale. Almonds will work instead of walnuts. And even though some produce (pineapples), whole grains (wild rice), nuts (pecans), and seafood (salmon) aren't really grown or harvested in the Mediterranean region, that doesn't mean you shouldn't happily swap them into recipes to make them your own.

One last note: Make this book messy! Dog-ear the pages and write notes in the margins. These recipes are a starting place to build your confidence in cooking the Mediterranean way, using what you have on hand and what tastes good to you and your family.

Now, let's get into the kitchen!

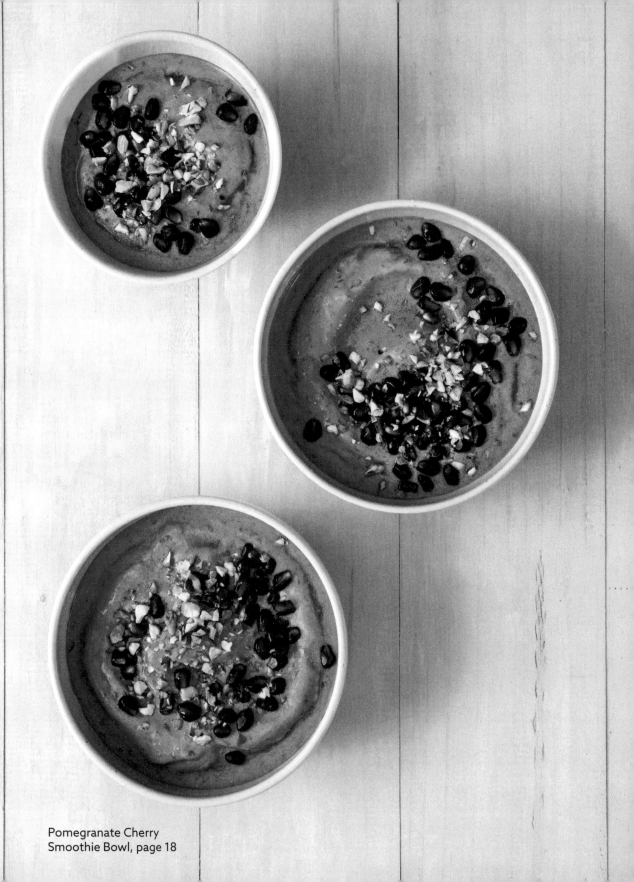

Pomegranate Cherry
Smoothie Bowl, page 18

TWO

Breakfast

GOOD morning! We've gathered up some of our favorite Mediterranean grains, fruits, and even veggies and are serving them to you for breakfast. These recipes range from a minutes-to-make Pomegranate Cherry Smoothie Bowl (page 18) to savory Marinara Eggs with Parsley (page 26). You'll be starting your day off right—with the nutrients your body needs after sleeping all night, and with the flavors your taste buds are craving.

Pomegranate Cherry Smoothie Bowl

SERVES

PREP TIME

GLUTEN-FREE, EGG-FREE, VEGETARIAN, HALF THE TIME

You won't miss the added sugar that often pops up in breakfast drinks with this Mediterranean-flavored smoothie bowl. The magical combo of pomegranate and cherry—along with a dash of cinnamon—provides all the natural sweetness you'll need in this creamy, frosty smoothie that's so thick, you can eat it with a spoon.

1 (16-ounce) bag frozen dark sweet cherries

1½ cups 2% plain Greek yogurt, plus more if needed

¾ cup pomegranate juice

⅓ cup 2% milk, plus more if needed

1 teaspoon vanilla extract

¾ teaspoon ground cinnamon

6 ice cubes

½ cup chopped pistachios

½ cup fresh pomegranate seeds

Per Serving Calories: 212; Total Fat: 7g; Saturated Fat: 3g; Cholesterol: 18mg; Sodium: 53mg; Total Carbohydrates: 35g; Fiber: 3g; Protein: 4g

1. Put the cherries, yogurt, pomegranate juice, milk, vanilla, cinnamon, and ice cubes in a blender. Purée until thoroughly mixed and smooth. You'll want the mixture a little thicker than your average smoothie, but not so thick you can't pour it. If the smoothie is too thick, add another few tablespoons of milk; if it's too thin, add another few tablespoons of yogurt.

2. Pour the smoothie into four bowls. Top each with 2 tablespoons of pistachios and 2 tablespoons of pomegranate seeds, and serve immediately.

Ingredient tip: You can buy packaged pomegranate seeds—also called arils—in the refrigerated produce section of your supermarket, but we'd also encourage you to try buying the whole fruit when they're in season. To avoid stains from pomegranate juice, try our trick of removing the seeds underwater: Fill a large bowl with water, submerge the pomegranate, and cut it into four sections. Working under the water, remove the seeds from the white membranes. The seeds will float to the top, and you can remove them with a strainer or slotted spoon.

Greek Yogurt Breakfast Parfaits with Roasted Grapes

GLUTEN-FREE, EGG-FREE, VEGETARIAN, 5 INGREDIENTS, ONE POT

SERVES

4

PREP TIME

5

COOK TIME

25

These roasted grapes are like little spoonfuls of grape jelly—but with zero added sugar. The oven caramelizes the natural sugars in the grapes until they become super sweet. Add roasted grapes to cereal, oatmeal, salads, whole grains, or peanut butter toast, or just eat them plain with a spoon.

1½ pounds seedless grapes (about 4 cups)

1 tablespoon extra-virgin olive oil

2 cups 2% plain Greek yogurt

½ cup chopped walnuts

4 teaspoons honey

Per Serving Calories: 300; Total Fat: 17g; Saturated Fat: 4g; Cholesterol: 16mg; Sodium: 59mg; Total Carbohydrates: 34g; Fiber: 2g; Protein: 7g

1. Place a large, rimmed baking sheet in the oven. Preheat the oven to 450°F with the pan inside.

2. Wash the grapes and remove from the stems. Dry on a clean kitchen towel, and put in a bowl. Drizzle with the oil, and toss to coat.

3. Carefully remove the hot pan from the oven, and pour the grapes onto the pan. Bake for 20 to 23 minutes, until slightly shriveled, stirring once halfway through. Remove the baking sheet from the oven and cool on a wire rack for 5 minutes.

4. While the grapes are cooling, assemble the parfaits by spooning the yogurt into four bowls or tall glasses. Top each bowl or glass with 2 tablespoons of walnuts and 1 teaspoon of honey.

5. When the grapes are slightly cooled, top each parfait with a quarter of the grapes. Scrape any accumulated sweet grape juice onto the parfaits and serve.

Prep tip: You can also roast the grapes still on their stems. Place them on the hot baking sheet, and use a basting brush to brush them with olive oil. After baking and cooling, remove the grapes from their stems, or serve them still on the stems on a cheese board like our Mediterranean Fruit, Veggie, and Cheese Board (page 30).

Mashed Chickpea, Feta, and Avocado Toast

NUT-FREE, EGG-FREE, VEGETARIAN, HALF THE TIME

Packed with fiber and protein, this Mediterranean version of avocado toast will keep you feeling full throughout the morning. It takes just minutes to mash up the avocado and beans, but you can make the spread the night before and then smear it onto your toast at breakfast time. You can also serve it in a bowl as a dip for an appetizer, or as a snack with raw veggies and pita wedges.

1 (15-ounce) can chickpeas, drained and rinsed

1 avocado, pitted

½ cup diced feta cheese (about 2 ounces)

2 teaspoons freshly squeezed lemon juice or 1 tablespoon orange juice

½ teaspoon freshly ground black pepper

4 pieces multigrain toast

2 teaspoons honey

1. Put the chickpeas in a large bowl. Scoop the avocado flesh into the bowl.

2. With a potato masher or large fork, mash the ingredients together until the mix has a spreadable consistency. It doesn't need to be totally smooth.

3. Add the feta, lemon juice, and pepper, and mix well.

4. Evenly divide the mash onto the four pieces of toast and spread with a knife. Drizzle with honey and serve.

Per Serving: Calories: 337; Total Fat: 13g; Saturated Fat: 4g; Cholesterol: 16mg; Sodium: 564mg; Total Carbohydrates: 43g; Fiber: 12g; Protein: 13g

Ingredient tip: If you can't find lower-sodium or no-salt-added canned beans, draining and rinsing a regular can of beans can still reduce the amount of sodium by around 40 percent.

Quickie Honey Nut Granola

GLUTEN-FREE, EGG-FREE, VEGETARIAN

There are many healthy-sounding granolas on the market, but they usually contain a lot of added sugar. You can make homemade granola in less than 30 minutes that is naturally sweetened by apricots, honey, cinnamon, and vanilla. Mix this granola into a plain whole-grain cereal like O-shaped oat rings or bran flakes, or layer it into our Greek Yogurt Breakfast Parfaits with Roasted Grapes (page 19).

2½ cups regular rolled oats

⅓ cup coarsely chopped almonds

⅛ teaspoon kosher or sea salt

½ teaspoon ground cinnamon

½ cup chopped dried apricots

2 tablespoons ground flaxseed

¼ cup honey

¼ cup extra-virgin olive oil

2 teaspoons vanilla extract

Per Serving Calories: 337; Total Fat: 17g; Saturated Fat: 2g; Cholesterol: 0mg; Sodium: 23mg; Total Carbohydrates: 42g; Fiber: 6g; Protein: 7g

1. Preheat the oven to 325°F. Line a large, rimmed baking sheet with parchment paper.

2. In a large skillet, combine the oats, almonds, salt, and cinnamon. Turn the heat to medium-high and cook, stirring often, to toast, about 6 minutes.

3. While the oat mixture is toasting, in a microwave-safe bowl, combine the apricots, flaxseed, honey, and oil. Microwave on high for about 1 minute, or until very hot and just beginning to bubble. (Or heat these ingredients in a small saucepan over medium heat for about 3 minutes.)

4. Stir the vanilla into the honey mixture, then pour it over the oat mixture in the skillet. Stir well.

5. Spread out the granola on the prepared baking sheet. Bake for 15 minutes, until lightly browned. Remove from the oven and cool completely.

6. Break the granola into small pieces, and store in an airtight container in the refrigerator for up to 2 weeks (if it lasts that long!).

Prep tip: When measuring nut butters, honey, maple syrup, or other sticky ingredients, first spray the measuring cup with nonstick cooking spray. Then when you pour (or dump) the sticky ingredients out, they will come right out.

Breakfast Polenta

SERVES

6

PREP TIME

5

COOK TIME

10

Back in the day, Deanna's mom would make cornmeal mush for breakfast with her 1970s avocado-green pressure cooker that sounded like it might explode at any moment. Luckily, since then, this recipe has evolved in both its cooking method and flavor profile. By using prepared polenta from a tube, you'll have a hot breakfast on the table in 15 minutes .

2 (18-ounce) tubes plain polenta

2¼ to 2½ cups 2% milk, divided

2 oranges, peeled and chopped

½ cup chopped pecans

¼ cup 2% plain Greek yogurt

8 teaspoons honey

Per Serving Calories: 234; Total Fat: 7g; Saturated Fat: 2g; Cholesterol: 5mg; Sodium: 438mg; Total Carbohydrates: 38mg; Fiber: 4g; Protein: 3g

1. Slice the polenta into rounds and place in a microwave-safe bowl. Heat in the microwave on high for 45 seconds.

2. Transfer the polenta to a large pot, and mash it with a potato masher or fork until coarsely mashed. Place the pot on the stove over medium heat.

3. In a medium, microwave-safe bowl, heat the milk in the microwave on high for 1 minute. Pour 2 cups of the warmed milk into the pot with the polenta, and stir with a whisk. Continue to stir and mash with the whisk, adding the remaining milk a few tablespoons at a time, until the polenta is fairly smooth and heated through, about 5 minutes. Remove from the stove.

4. Divide the polenta among four serving bowls. Top each bowl with one-quarter of the oranges, 2 tablespoons of pecans, 1 tablespoon of yogurt, and 2 teaspoons of honey before serving.

Ingredient tip: Instead of the cooked tubed polenta, you can buy medium-ground or coarsely ground cornmeal, which both have the right consistency to make traditional Italian polenta but take longer to cook. Look for the phrase "stone-ground whole corn," which indicates a whole grain. Follow the directions on the package, using a mixture of half milk and half water for the liquid.

Baked Ricotta with Pears

If you like ricotta-style cheesecake, you'll love this dessert for breakfast. It's a portion-controlled, healthier twist that's made with less sugar but still has that decadent, creamy taste. This protein-rich breakfast calls for whole-milk ricotta cheese for the ultimate appeal, but if you want to cut a few more calories, use the part-skim version. The white whole wheat flour we recommend for this recipe is still whole wheat. Instead of the traditional dark brown whole wheat flour, white whole wheat flour is made with a different type of wheat that is lighter in color with a milder flavor and a softer texture. It's fairly easy to find in the baking aisle of the supermarket.

Nonstick cooking spray

1 (16-ounce) container whole-milk ricotta cheese

2 large eggs

¼ cup white whole-wheat flour or whole-wheat pastry flour

1 tablespoon sugar

1 teaspoon vanilla extract

¼ teaspoon ground nutmeg

1 pear, cored and diced

2 tablespoons water

1 tablespoon honey

1. Preheat the oven to 400°F. Spray four 6-ounce ramekins with nonstick cooking spray.

2. In a large bowl, beat together the ricotta, eggs, flour, sugar, vanilla, and nutmeg. Spoon into the ramekins. Bake for 22 to 25 minutes, or until the ricotta is just about set. Remove from the oven and cool slightly on racks.

3. While the ricotta is baking, in a small saucepan over medium heat, simmer the pear in the water for 10 minutes, until slightly softened. Remove from the heat, and stir in the honey.

4. Serve the ricotta ramekins topped with the warmed pear.

Per Serving Calories: 312; Total Fat: 17g; Saturated Fat: 10g; Cholesterol: 163mg; Sodium: 130mg; Total Carbohydrates: 23g; Fiber: 2g; Protein: 17g

Prep tip: If you don't have ramekins, use a baking pan and increase the baking time by 10 minutes. You can also heat the pear in the microwave instead of on the stove top. Place the pear and water in a microwave-safe glass bowl and cook on high for 3 minutes. Stir in the honey.

Mediterranean Fruit Bulgur Breakfast Bowl

EGG-FREE, VEGETARIAN, ONE POT

Bulgur is whole wheat that has been partially cooked and then dried. Traditionally it's used in savory recipes like the classic tabbouleh salad (see our Stuffed Tomatoes with Tabbouleh on page 124). When it's cooked in milk, it becomes thick and creamy, making it an ideal hot breakfast cereal. Figs are so sweet you won't need to add any sugar to this recipe.

1½ cups uncooked bulgur

2 cups 2% milk

1 cup water

½ teaspoon ground cinnamon

2 cups frozen (or fresh, pitted) dark sweet cherries

8 dried (or fresh) figs, chopped

½ cup chopped almonds

¼ cup loosely packed fresh mint, chopped

Warm 2% milk, for serving (optional)

Per Serving Calories: 301; Total Fat: 6g; Saturated Fat: 1g; Cholesterol: 7mg; Sodium: 40mg; Total Carbohydrates: 57g; Fiber: 9g; Protein: 9g

1. In a medium saucepan, combine the bulgur, milk, water, and cinnamon. Stir once, then bring just to a boil. Cover, reduce the heat to medium-low, and simmer for 10 minutes or until the liquid is absorbed.

2. Turn off the heat, but keep the pan on the stove, and stir in the frozen cherries (no need to thaw), figs, and almonds. Stir well, cover for 1 minute, and let the hot bulgur thaw the cherries and partially hydrate the figs. Stir in the mint.

3. Scoop into serving bowls. Serve with warm milk, if desired. You can also serve it chilled.

Prep tip: Dried fruit can be cumbersome to chop; the fruit pieces can stick to the knife, forcing you to stop often to remove them. To prevent this, spray your knife with nonstick cooking spray to slice easily through dried fruit.

Scrambled Eggs with Goat Cheese and Roasted Peppers

NUT-FREE, DAIRY-FREE, GLUTEN-FREE, VEGETARIAN,
5 INGREDIENTS, ONE POT, HALF THE TIME

SERVES

4

PREP
TIME

5

COOK
TIME

10

This scrambled egg dish is quick enough to serve on a weekday morning—and it's a protein-packed way to start the day. Maintaining muscle mass, especially after age 30, keeps our bodies strong and may prevent injuries and weight gain. Most importantly, eggs, peppers, goat cheese, and mint are a delicious combination to wake up to.

1½ teaspoons
extra-virgin olive oil

1 cup chopped bell
peppers, any color (about
1 medium pepper)

2 garlic cloves, minced
(about 1 teaspoon)

6 large eggs

¼ teaspoon kosher
or sea salt

2 tablespoons water

½ cup crumbled goat
cheese (about 2 ounces)

2 tablespoons loosely
packed chopped fresh mint

Per Serving Calories: 201;
Total Fat: 15g; Saturated Fat: 6g;
Cholesterol: 294mg; Sodium:
176mg; Total Carbohydrates: 5g;
Fiber: 2g; Protein: 15g

1. In a large skillet over medium-high heat, heat the oil. Add the peppers and cook for 5 minutes, stirring occasionally. Add the garlic and cook for 1 minute.

2. While the peppers are cooking, in a medium bowl, whisk together the eggs, salt, and water.

3. Turn the heat down to medium-low. Pour the egg mixture over the peppers. Let the eggs cook undisturbed for 1 to 2 minutes, until they begin to set on the bottom. Sprinkle with the goat cheese.

4. Cook the eggs for about 1 to 2 more minutes, stirring slowly, until the eggs are soft-set and custardy. (They will continue to cook off the stove from the residual heat in the pan.)

5. Top with the fresh mint and serve.

Prep tip: To prevent tough scrambled eggs, cook them low and slow. If you cook on an electric stove, give your burners a few minutes to cool down when you turn down the heat, then place the skillet back on when the burner is truly at a medium-low heat.

Marinara Eggs with Parsley

NUT-FREE, GLUTEN-FREE, VEGETARIAN, 5 INGREDIENTS, ONE POT

SERVES

6

PREP TIME

5

COOK TIME

15

While this pan of eggs makes an impressive brunch for guests, it's also a great simple breakfast for the family. And in reality, Serena serves it most often for dinner. Here the parsley not only adds a fresh taste and a pop of color against the bright tomatoes and eggs, but it also adds big nutrition.

1 tablespoon extra-virgin olive oil

1 cup chopped onion (about ½ medium onion)

2 garlic cloves, minced (about 1 teaspoon)

2 (14.5-ounce) cans Italian diced tomatoes, undrained, no salt added

6 large eggs

½ cup chopped fresh flat-leaf (Italian) parsley

Crusty Italian bread and grated Parmesan or Romano cheese, for serving (optional)

Per Serving Calories: 122; Total Fat: 7g; Saturated Fat: 2g; Cholesterol: 186mg; Sodium: 207mg; Total Carbohydrates: 7g; Fiber: 1g; Protein: 7g

1. In a large skillet over medium-high heat, heat the oil. Add the onion and cook for 5 minutes, stirring occasionally. Add the garlic and cook for 1 minute.

2. Pour the tomatoes with their juices over the onion mixture and cook until bubbling, 2 to 3 minutes. While waiting for the tomato mixture to bubble, crack one egg into a small custard cup or coffee mug.

3. When the tomato mixture bubbles, lower the heat to medium. Then use a large spoon to make six indentations in the tomato mixture. Gently pour the first cracked egg into one indentation and repeat, cracking the remaining eggs, one at a time, into the custard cup and pouring one into each indentation. Cover the skillet and cook for 6 to 7 minutes, or until the eggs are done to your liking (about 6 minutes for soft-cooked, 7 minutes for harder cooked).

4. Top with the parsley, and serve with the bread and grated cheese, if desired.

Ingredient tip: A can of Italian diced tomatoes is a convenient ingredient to keep in your pantry and typically contains any combination of onion, garlic, basil, and oregano. Look for cans with only 6 grams or less of sugar and no salt added.

Italian Breakfast Bruschetta

NUT-FREE

SERVES

4

PREP TIME

10

COOK TIME

20

Upgrade your typical bacon and eggs breakfast with this hearty toast topper featuring scrambled eggs, prosciutto, and broccoli rabe. Broccoli rabe can be somewhat bitter if not cooked correctly, so boiling before sautéing is important.

¼ teaspoon kosher or sea salt

6 cups broccoli rabe, stemmed and chopped (about 1 bunch)

1 tablespoon extra-virgin olive oil

2 garlic cloves, minced (about 1 teaspoon)

1 ounce prosciutto, cut or torn into ½-inch pieces

¼ teaspoon crushed red pepper

Nonstick cooking spray

3 large eggs

1 tablespoon 2% milk

¼ teaspoon freshly ground black pepper

4 teaspoons grated Parmesan or Pecorino Romano cheese

1 garlic clove, halved

8 (¾-inch-thick) slices baguette-style whole-grain bread or 4 slices larger Italian-style whole-grain bread

1. Bring a large stockpot of water to a boil. Add the salt and broccoli rabe, and boil for 2 minutes. Drain in a colander.

2. In a large skillet over medium heat, heat the oil. Add the garlic, prosciutto, and crushed red pepper, and cook for 2 minutes, stirring often. Add the broccoli rabe and cook for an additional 3 minutes, stirring a few times. Transfer to a bowl and set aside.

3. Place the skillet back on the stove over low heat and coat with nonstick cooking spray.

4. In a small bowl, whisk together the eggs, milk, and pepper. Pour into the skillet. Stir and cook until the eggs are soft scrambled, 3 to 5 minutes. Add the broccoli rabe mixture back to the skillet along with the cheese. Stir and cook for about 1 minute, until heated through. Remove from the heat.

5. Toast the bread, then rub the cut sides of the garlic clove halves onto one side of each slice of the toast. (Save the garlic for another recipe.) Spoon the egg mixture onto each piece of toast and serve.

Ingredient tip: You can swap in chopped spinach for the broccoli rabe. Skip the boiling and just cook the spinach in the skillet for 2 to 3 minutes, as described in step 2.

Per Serving Calories: 216; Total Fat: 9g; Saturated Fat: 2g; Cholesterol: 145mg; Sodium: 522mg; Total Carbohydrates: 20g; Fiber: 5g; Protein: 13g

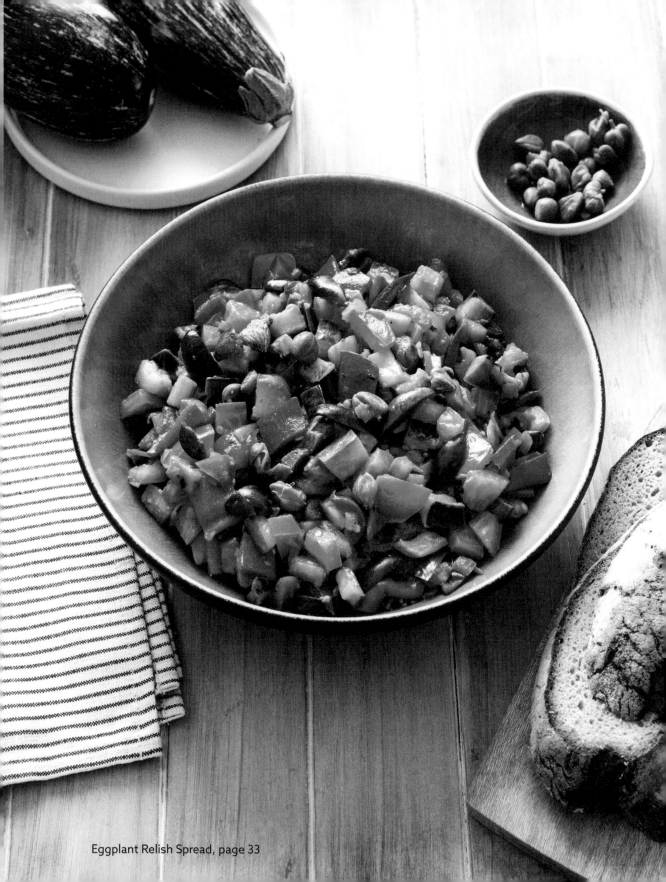

Eggplant Relish Spread, page 33

THREE

Small Plates and Snacks

WHILE many diets ditch the snacks, we think they are an important part of a nutritionally sound eating plan. They help you keep hunger in check and prevent you from becoming ravenous or making less-than-healthy choices at your next meal. People who live a Mediterranean lifestyle rarely snack on anything more than fruit or a handful of nuts—and that's fine if that's what you crave. But for the times when you want something a little bit more—like tangy Lemony Garlic Hummus (page 31) or boldly flavored Crunchy Orange-Thyme Chickpeas (page 36)—and you want it sooner rather than later, we have you covered with eight recipes for satisfying small bites and munchies.

Mediterranean Fruit, Veggie, and Cheese Board

SERVES

4

PREP TIME

15

NUT-FREE, GLUTEN-FREE, EGG-FREE, HALF THE TIME

This is less of a recipe and more of a formula to follow for the portions and types of ingredients you could include in this fancy-sounding but simple-to-assemble snack plate. Use small bowls or ramekins for runny or delicate ingredients, like roasted red peppers, olives, and berries. Or turn this into a party appetizer by doubling the amounts for a crowd.

2 cups sliced fruits, such as apples, pears, plums, or peaches

2 cups finger-food fruits, such as berries, cherries, grapes, or figs

2 cups raw vegetables cut into sticks, such as carrots, celery, broccoli, cauliflower, or whole cherry tomatoes

1 cup cured, canned, or jarred vegetables, such as roasted peppers or artichoke hearts, or ½ cup olives

1 cup cubed cheese, such as goat cheese, Gorgonzola, feta, Manchego, or Asiago (about 4 ounces)

1. Wash all the fresh produce and cut into slices or bite-size pieces, as described in the ingredients list.

2. Arrange all the ingredients on a wooden board or serving tray. Include small spoons for items like the berries and olives, and a fork or knife for the cheeses. Serve with small plates and napkins.

Prep tip: If your wooden cutting boards aren't big enough or are beat-up looking (like Deanna's), cover a large, rimmed baking sheet with parchment paper. The contrast of the paper makes all the colorful ingredients pop, and it also makes cleanup super easy.

Per Serving Calories: 213; Total Fat: 9g; Saturated Fat: 4g; Cholesterol: 25mg; Sodium: 466mg; Total Carbohydrates: 30g; Fiber: 5g; Protein: 6g

Lemony Garlic Hummus

GLUTEN-FREE, VEGAN, 5 INGREDIENTS, HALF THE TIME

SERVES

6

PREP
TIME

5

We realize you can buy hummus in the store. But homemade is so much better, and it's easy to make! Peanut butter is the surprising ingredient—we use it because it's more common and budget-friendly than tahini (sesame paste), the traditional hummus ingredient. The subtle nutty flavor of the peanut butter blends perfectly with the other ingredients to create a super-quick dip, spread, or sandwich filler.

1 (15-ounce) can chickpeas, drained, liquid reserved

3 tablespoons freshly squeezed lemon juice (from about 1 large lemon)

2 tablespoons peanut butter

3 tablespoons extra-virgin olive oil, divided

2 garlic cloves

¼ teaspoon kosher or sea salt (optional)

Raw veggies or whole-grain crackers, for serving (optional)

Per Serving Calories: 165; Total Fat: 11g; Saturated Fat: 2g; Cholesterol: 0mg; Sodium: 348mg; Total Carbohydrates: 14g; Fiber: 4g; Protein: 5g

1. In the bowl of a food processor, combine the chickpeas and 2 tablespoons of the reserved chickpea liquid with the lemon juice, peanut butter, 2 tablespoons of oil, and the garlic. Process the mixture for 1 minute. Scrape down the sides of the bowl with a rubber spatula. Process for 1 more minute, or until smooth.

2. Put in a serving bowl, drizzle with the remaining 1 tablespoon of olive oil, sprinkle with the salt, if using, and serve with veggies or crackers, if desired.

Prep tip: The key to light, airy hummus is to add some chickpea liquid, also known as *aquafaba*. While we usually recommend draining and rinsing canned beans to remove more sodium, for this recipe, save that liquid gold to make your hummus beyond delicious.

Romesco Dip

SERVES

10

PREP TIME

10

This flavorful recipe is based on a traditional sauce from the Catalonia area of Spain. With just a few whirls of the blender you'll have an instant appetizer, a topping for chicken or seafood, a sauce for pasta, or a base for vegetable soup.

1 (12-ounce) jar roasted red peppers, drained

1 (14.5-ounce) can diced tomatoes, undrained

½ cup dry-roasted almonds

2 garlic cloves

2 teaspoons red wine vinegar

1 teaspoon smoked paprika or ½ teaspoon cayenne pepper

¼ teaspoon kosher or sea salt

¼ teaspoon freshly ground black pepper

¼ cup extra-virgin olive oil

2/3 cup torn, day-old bread or toast (about 2 slices)

Assortment of sliced raw vegetables such as carrots, celery, cucumber, green beans, and bell peppers, for serving

1. In a high-powered blender or food processor, combine the roasted peppers, tomatoes and their juices, almonds, garlic, vinegar, smoked paprika, salt, and pepper.

2. Begin puréeing the ingredients on medium speed, and slowly drizzle in the oil with the blender running. Continue to purée until the dip is thoroughly mixed.

3. Add the bread and purée.

4. Serve with raw vegetables for dipping, or store in a jar with a lid for up to one week in the refrigerator.

Ingredient tip: Look for fire-roasted canned tomatoes in the store to add even more flavor to this dip. To make it gluten-free, simply omit the bread.

Per Serving Calories:107; Total Fat: 9g; Saturated Fat: 1g; Cholesterol: 0mg; Sodium: 216mg; Total Carbohydrates: 6g; Fiber: 3g; Protein: 2g

Eggplant Relish Spread

NUT-FREE, GLUTEN-FREE, VEGAN, ONE POT

SERVES
6

PREP TIME
10

COOK TIME
20

Also known as caponata, this Sicilian condiment is sweet, sour, savory, and oh so delicious! It's also a great way to change the minds of people who say they don't like eggplant. Spread it on crusty whole-grain bread, spoon it over scrambled eggs, have it with grilled chicken, or serve it in a bowl on the Mediterranean Fruit, Veggie, and Cheese Board (page 30).

2 tablespoons extra-virgin olive oil

1 cup finely chopped onion (about ½ medium onion)

1 garlic clove, minced (about ½ teaspoon)

1 large globe eggplant, cut into ½-inch cubes (about 5 cups)

¼ teaspoon kosher or sea salt

1 (12-ounce) jar roasted red peppers, chopped

1½ cups chopped fresh tomatoes

½ cup balsamic or red wine vinegar

½ cup capers or chopped olives

Per Serving Calories: 101; Total Fat: 5g; Saturated Fat: 1g; Cholesterol: 0mg; Sodium 396mg; Total Carbohydrates: 13g; Fiber: 5g; Protein: 2g

1. In a large skillet over medium heat, heat the oil.

2. Add the onion and cook for 4 minutes, stirring occasionally. Add the garlic and cook for 1 minute, stirring often. Turn up the heat to medium-high, and add the eggplant and salt. Cook for 5 minutes, stirring occasionally.

3. Add the peppers, tomatoes, and vinegar, stir, and cover. Cook for 10 minutes, stirring every minute or so to prevent everything from sticking. If it looks like it's starting to stick and burn, turn down the heat to medium and add 1 tablespoon of water.

4. Remove from the heat, stir in the capers, and let sit for a few minutes to let the liquid absorb. Stir and serve, or store in a covered jar in the refrigerator for up to 10 days. It tastes even better the day after you make it!

Ingredient tip: In the past, salting and then draining raw eggplant slices in a colander for 30 minutes would help remove some of the vegetable's bitter flavor. However, today, the majority of eggplants—like the large purple variety—are cultivated to be less bitter, so you can skip this step.

Honey-Rosemary Almonds

SERVES

6

PREP TIME

5

COOK TIME

10

As dietitians, we recommend nuts as the ideal snack because they are the right combination of better-for-you fats and protein—both of which will keep you feeling fuller longer. As food lovers, we recommend them because from almonds to pistachios, there's a yummy nut for everyone. These sweet and savory almonds can be whipped up in minutes and are a delicious addition to salads or whole-grain dishes.

1 cup raw, whole, shelled almonds

1 tablespoon minced fresh rosemary

¼ teaspoon kosher or sea salt

1 tablespoon honey

Nonstick cooking spray

Per serving Calories: 149; Total Fat: 12g; Saturated Fat: 0g; Cholesterol: 0mg; Sodium: 78mg; Total Carbohydrates: 8g; Fiber: 3g; Protein: 5g

1. In a large skillet over medium heat, combine the almonds, rosemary, and salt. Stir frequently for 1 minute.

2. Drizzle in the honey and cook for another 3 to 4 minutes, stirring frequently, until the almonds are coated and just starting to darken around the edges.

3. Remove from the heat. Using a spatula, spread the almonds onto a pan coated with nonstick cooking spray. Cool for 10 minutes or so. Break up the almonds before serving.

Ingredient tip: Experiment with different nuts in this recipe, such as walnuts, pecans, or peanuts, or other herbs and spices, like thyme, chili powder, or cinnamon.

Fig-Pecan Energy Bites

DAIRY-FREE, GLUTEN-FREE, EGG-FREE, VEGETARIAN

SERVES

6

PREP
TIME

20

These two-bite snack balls are just the right amount of sweet goodness. While you can use your food processor to quickly whizz together the ingredients, we don't bother. The process of chopping the figs and pecans by hand and mixing it together takes only about 15 minutes (and gives you a bonus arm workout!).

¾ cup diced dried
figs (6 to 8)

½ cup chopped pecans

¼ cup rolled oats
(old-fashioned or
quick oats)

2 tablespoons ground
flaxseed or wheat germ
(flaxseed for gluten-free)

2 tablespoons powdered
or regular peanut butter

2 tablespoons honey

Per Serving Calories: 157; Total
Fat: 6g; Saturated Fat: 1g; Choles-
terol: 0mg; Sodium: 28mg; Total
Carbohydrates: 26g; Fiber: 4g;
Protein: 3g

1. In a medium bowl, mix together the figs, pecans, oats, flaxseed, and peanut butter. Drizzle with the honey, and mix everything together. A wooden spoon works well to press the figs and nuts into the honey and powdery ingredients. (If you're using regular peanut butter instead of powdered, the dough will be stickier to handle, so freeze the dough for 5 minutes before making the bites.)

2. Divide the dough evenly into four sections in the bowl. Dampen your hands with water—but don't get them too wet or the dough will stick to them. Using your hands, roll three bites out of each of the four sections of dough, making 12 total energy bites.

3. Enjoy immediately or chill in the freezer for 5 minutes to firm up the bites before serving. The bites can be stored in a sealed container in the refrigerator for up to 1 week.

Prep tip: Many recipes for fruit and nut snack balls call for refrigerating the dough for at least 30 minutes, to make shaping the balls easier. You can skip this step if you plan ahead and refrigerate all the ingredients (except the honey) for at least 15 minutes before mixing.

Crunchy Orange-Thyme Chickpeas

NUT-FREE, GLUTEN-FREE, VEGAN, 5 INGREDIENTS, ONE POT

SERVES

4

PREP TIME

5

COOK TIME

20

These snackable chickpeas are absolutely addictive straight out of the oven. After cooling, they get a bit chewy on the inside—but they're still just as tasty. If you make these ahead of time, warm them up again with a brief blast of heat for about 1 minute or so under your broiler (watch carefully to prevent burning) before serving.

1 (15-ounce) can chickpeas, drained and rinsed

2 teaspoons extra-virgin olive oil

¼ teaspoon dried thyme or ½ teaspoon chopped fresh thyme leaves

⅛ teaspoon kosher or sea salt

Zest of ½ orange (about ½ teaspoon)

Per Serving Calories: 128; Total Fat: 4g; Saturated Fat: 1g; Cholesterol: 0mg; Sodium: 299mg; Total Carbohydrates: 18g; Fiber: 5g; Protein: 5g

1. Preheat the oven to 450°F.

2. Spread the chickpeas on a clean kitchen towel, and rub gently until dry.

3. Spread the chickpeas on a large, rimmed baking sheet. Drizzle with the oil, and sprinkle with the thyme and salt. Using a Microplane or citrus zester, zest about half of the orange over the chickpeas. Mix well using your hands.

4. Bake for 10 minutes, then open the oven door and, using an oven mitt, give the baking sheet a quick shake. (Do not remove the sheet from the oven.) Bake for 10 minutes more. Taste the chickpeas (carefully!). If they are golden but you think they could be a bit crunchier, bake for 3 minutes more before serving.

Ingredient tip: Change up the flavor combination of this fun snack. Try ¼ teaspoon each of cumin and lime zest, or try ¼ teaspoon each of curry powder and ground ginger. Serena's favorite combo is ¼ teaspoon each of unsweetened cocoa powder and smoked paprika.

Sesame-Thyme Mano'ushe Flatbread

NUT-FREE, VEGAN, 5 INGREDIENTS, HALF THE TIME, ONE POT

SERVES

6

PREP TIME

5

COOK TIME

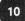
10

Mano'ushe is a Lebanese-style flatbread generously topped with olive oil and seasoned with za'atar. This pizza-like bread is typically bought at local bakeries and eaten on the go for breakfast or as a snack. In this recipe, we use refrigerated whole-wheat pizza dough, found in supermarkets, but if you don't feel like rolling out the dough, you can also use whole-wheat pita or lavash bread.

Nonstick cooking spray

1 (16-ounce) bag whole-wheat pizza dough or 3 (6-inch) whole-wheat pita breads

3 tablespoons dried thyme

3 tablespoons sesame seeds

3 tablespoons extra-virgin olive oil

¼ teaspoon kosher or sea salt

Per Serving Calories: 175; Total Fat: 10g; Saturated Fat: 2g; Cholesterol: 0mg; Sodium: 249mg; Total Carbohydrates: 20g; Fiber: 3g; Protein: 4g

1. Preheat the oven to 450°F. Spray a large, rimmed baking sheet with nonstick cooking spray.

2. Divide the dough into three equal balls. On a floured surface, roll each dough ball with a rolling pin into a 6-inch circle. Place all three dough circles (or pita breads) on the baking sheet.

3. In a small bowl, whisk together the thyme, sesame seeds, oil, and salt. With a pastry brush or spoon, brush the oil onto the three dough circles (or pita breads) until it's all used up.

4. Bake the dough circles for 10 minutes, or until the edges just start to brown and crisp and the oil is cooked into the dough. If using pita rounds, bake them for only 5 minutes. Remove the flatbreads from the oven, cut each circle in half, and serve.

Ingredient tip: Za'atar is actually an herb, but it's more commonly known as a spice blend, typically made up of sesame seeds, salt, and other herbs such as thyme, oregano, marjoram, and sumac. If you buy a packaged za'atar spice blend, use 6 tablespoons of it instead of the thyme, sesame seeds, and salt in this recipe.

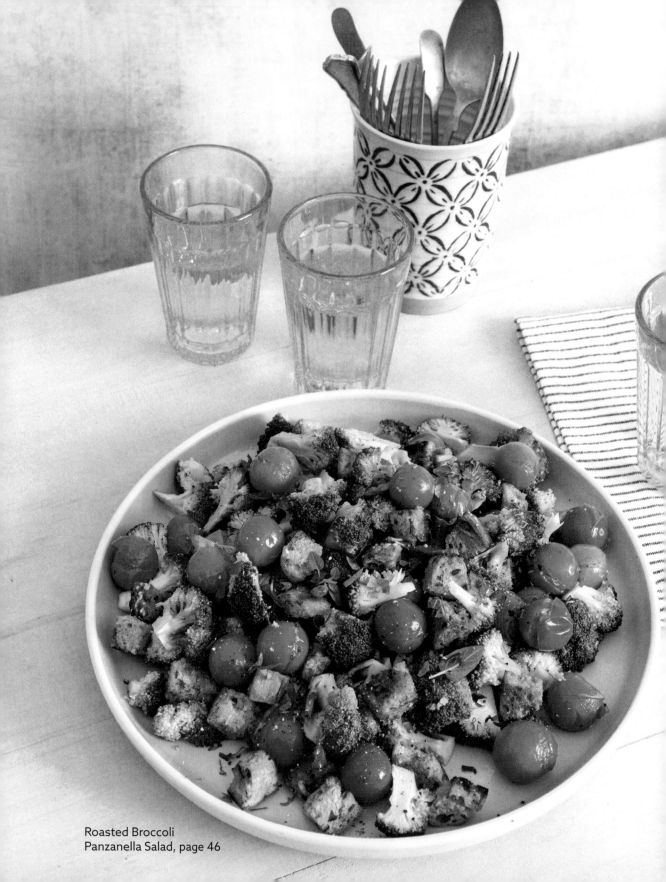

Roasted Broccoli
Panzanella Salad, page 46

FOUR

Salads and Soups

WHY settle for limp side salads or high-sodium soups when you can whip up good-for-you and great-tasting dishes such as Roasted Broccoli Panzanella Salad (page 46) and Paella Soup (page 52) in a half hour or less? All of our salads, from Melon Caprese Salad (page 42) to Easy Italian Orange and Celery Salad (page 41), rely on robust yet familiar ingredients to deliver mealtime gratification. As for our soup recipes, we take advantage of simple yet powerful flavor bombs like rosemary and mushrooms, along with cooking techniques like roasting and puréeing, to achieve maximum flavor using minimal salt.

Pistachio-Parmesan Kale-Arugula Salad

SERVES

6

PREP TIME

20

GLUTEN-FREE, EGG-FREE, VEGETARIAN

We get it. Raw kale can be a turnoff because of its tough texture and biting taste. Massaging the leaves with a dressing and letting it sit for about 10 minutes starts to break down the fibrous leaves, resulting in milder, more tender kale. If you want to skip the massaging, look for baby kale, which has more delicate leaves.

6 cups raw kale, center ribs removed and discarded, leaves coarsely chopped

¼ cup extra-virgin olive oil

2 tablespoons freshly squeezed lemon juice (from about 1 small lemon)

½ teaspoon smoked paprika

2 cups arugula

⅓ cup unsalted shelled pistachios

6 tablespoons grated Parmesan or Pecorino Romano cheese

1. In a large salad bowl, combine the kale, oil, lemon juice, and smoked paprika. With your hands, gently massage the leaves for about 15 seconds or so, until all are thoroughly coated. Let the kale sit for 10 minutes.

2. When you're ready to serve, gently mix in the arugula and pistachios. Divide the salad among six serving bowls, sprinkle 1 tablespoon of grated cheese over each, and serve.

Ingredient tip: Save some dollars and buy pistachios in their shells. Sure, it takes a few minutes to remove the shells, but they're less expensive than the shelled variety, and in some cases even fresher tasting.

Per Serving Calories: 150; Total Fat: 12g; Saturated Fat: 2g; Cholesterol: 5mg; Sodium: 189mg; Total Carbohydrates: 8g; Fiber: 2g; Protein: 5g

Easy Italian Orange and Celery Salad

SERVES

6

PREP TIME

15

~~~~~~

NUT-FREE, GLUTEN-FREE, 5 INGREDIENTS, VEGAN, HALF THE TIME

~~~~~~

This salad is made with just a few ingredients that you probably have on hand—including entire celery stalks, so don't toss those tasty celery leaves. It's a pretty side dish to bring to any gathering. Serena likes to pack the salad and dressing separately. When you arrive at your destination, arrange on a serving platter and drizzle on the dressing.

3 celery stalks, including leaves, sliced diagonally into ½-inch slices

2 large oranges, peeled and sliced into rounds

½ cup green olives (or any variety)

¼ cup sliced red onion (about ¼ onion)

1 tablespoon extra-virgin olive oil

1 tablespoon olive brine

1 tablespoon freshly squeezed lemon or orange juice (from ½ small lemon or 1 orange round)

¼ teaspoon kosher or sea salt

¼ teaspoon freshly ground black pepper

1. Place the celery, oranges, olives, and onion on a large serving platter or in a shallow, wide bowl.

2. In a small bowl, whisk together the oil, olive brine, and lemon juice. Pour over the salad, sprinkle with salt and pepper, and serve.

Ingredient tip: Instead of the orange rounds in this salad, you can swap in peeled and sectioned clementines or canned mandarin oranges in juice that have been drained.

Per Serving Calories: 65; Total Fat: 4g; Saturated Fat: 0g; Cholesterol: 0mg; Sodium: 258mg; Total Carbohydrates: 9g; Fiber: 3g; Protein: 2g

Melon Caprese Salad

NUT-FREE, GLUTEN-FREE, EGG-FREE, VEGETARIAN

SERVES

6

PREP TIME

20

Here we give a refreshing twist to the classic caprese salad by adding ripe, juicy watermelon and cantaloupe. When the warmer weather hits, this is Deanna's go-to side dish for picnics, pool parties, or any summer celebration—and it always gets rave reviews. You may be surprised to see fruit paired with tomatoes, mozzarella, and basil, but it totally works (and tomatoes are a fruit, after all).

1 cantaloupe, quartered and seeded

½ small seedless watermelon

1 cup grape tomatoes

2 cups fresh mozzarella balls (about 8 ounces)

⅓ cup fresh basil or mint leaves, torn into small pieces

2 tablespoons extra-virgin olive oil

1 tablespoon balsamic vinegar

¼ teaspoon freshly ground black pepper

¼ teaspoon kosher or sea salt

Per Serving Calories: 218; Total Fat: 13g; Saturated Fat: 6g; Cholesterol: 27mg; Sodium: 296mg; Total Carbohydrates: 17g; Fiber: 1g; Protein: 10g

1. Using a melon baller or a metal, teaspoon-size measuring spoon, scoop balls out of the cantaloupe. You should get about 2½ to 3 cups from one cantaloupe. (If you prefer, cut the melon into bite-size pieces instead of making balls.) Put them in a large colander over a large serving bowl.

2. Using the same method, ball or cut the watermelon into bite-size pieces; you should get about 2 cups. Put the watermelon balls in the colander with the cantaloupe.

3. Let the fruit drain for 10 minutes. Pour the juice from the bowl into a container to refrigerate and save for drinking or adding to smoothies. Wipe the bowl dry, and put in the cut fruit.

4. Add the tomatoes, mozzarella, basil, oil, vinegar, pepper, and salt to the fruit mixture. Gently mix until everything is incorporated and serve.

Prep tip: If you want to make this recipe a day ahead, prepare the salad through step 3. Cover and refrigerate. Before serving, drain the fruit again for about 5 minutes. Add it back into the serving bowl, then toss it with the remaining ingredients.

Chopped Greek Antipasto Salad

NUT-FREE, GLUTEN-FREE, EGG-FREE, VEGETARIAN

SERVES

6

PREP TIME

20

Dietitian's confession: Deanna is not the biggest salad lover—at least, not salads that are almost all leafy greens. That's why she prefers a generous chopped salad where the mix-ins feature prominently rather than getting lost in a bowl of lettuce. Traditional Greek flavors—lemon and oregano—shine in this fragrant dressing, which you can also drizzle over baked or grilled fish, shrimp, or chicken.

For the salad

1 head Bibb lettuce or ½ head romaine lettuce, chopped (about 2½ cups)

¼ cup loosely packed chopped basil leaves

1 (15-ounce) can chickpeas, drained and rinsed

1 (14-ounce) can artichoke hearts, drained and halved

1 pint grape tomatoes, halved (about 1½ cups)

1 seedless cucumber, peeled and chopped (about 1½ cups)

½ cup cubed feta cheese (about 2 ounces)

1 (2.25-ounce) can sliced black olives (about ½ cup)

For the dressing

3 tablespoons extra-virgin olive oil

1 tablespoon red wine vinegar

1 tablespoon freshly squeezed lemon juice (from about ½ small lemon)

1 tablespoon chopped fresh oregano or ½ teaspoon dried oregano

1 teaspoon honey

¼ teaspoon freshly ground black pepper

Per Serving Calories: 226; Total Fat: 13g; Saturated Fat: 3g; Cholesterol: 11mg; Sodium: 545mg; Total Carbohydrates: 23g; Fiber: 8g; Protein: 8g

CONTINUES NEXT PAGE

To make the salad

In a medium bowl, toss the lettuce and basil together. Spread out on a large serving platter or in a large salad bowl. Arrange the chickpeas, artichoke hearts, tomatoes, cucumber, feta, and olives in piles next to each other on top of the lettuce layer.

To make the dressing

In a small pitcher or bowl, whisk together the oil, vinegar, lemon juice, oregano, honey, and pepper. Serve on the side with the salad, or drizzle over all the ingredients right before serving.

Prep tip: Take this dressing to the next level and make a quick oregano oil infusion. Put the oil and oregano in a small skillet over medium-low heat. Let it cook for 5 minutes, stirring occasionally. Remove from the heat and strain through a fine mesh strainer. Try this method with other herbs and spices, such as cumin, smoked paprika, rosemary, or minced garlic.

Mediterranean Potato Salad

NUT-FREE, GLUTEN-FREE, VEGAN, ONE POT

SERVES

6

PREP
TIME

10

COOK
TIME
20

Serena spent her honeymoon in Greece, so the combination of olives, lemons, oregano, and mint is near and dear to her heart. These aromatic ingredients are grown in regions all around the Mediterranean Sea. Serena likes to make this vacation-inspired potato salad all year round. It's equally delicious served chilled at a summer picnic, at room temperature in the autumn, or warm in the winter.

2 pounds Yukon Gold baby potatoes, cut into 1-inch cubes

3 tablespoons freshly squeezed lemon juice (from about 1 medium lemon)

3 tablespoons extra-virgin olive oil

1 tablespoon olive brine

¼ teaspoon kosher or sea salt

1 (2.25-ounce) can sliced olives (about ½ cup)

1 cup sliced celery (about 2 stalks) or fennel

2 tablespoons chopped fresh oregano

2 tablespoons torn fresh mint

Per Serving Calories: 175; Total Fat: 7g; Saturated Fat: 1g; Cholesterol: 0mg; Sodium: 98mg; Total Carbohydrates: 27g; Fiber: 4g; Protein: 3g

1. In a medium saucepan, cover the potatoes with cold water until the waterline is one inch above the potatoes. Set over high heat, bring the potatoes to a boil, then turn down the heat to medium-low. Simmer for 12 to 15 minutes, until the potatoes are just fork tender.

2. While the potatoes are cooking, in a small bowl, whisk together the lemon juice, oil, olive brine, and salt.

3. Drain the potatoes in a colander and transfer to a serving bowl. Immediately pour about 3 tablespoons of the dressing over the potatoes. Gently mix in the olives and celery.

4. Before serving, gently mix in the oregano, mint, and the remaining dressing.

Prep tip: The trick to bold—not bland—potato salad is to flavor the hot potatoes immediately after draining the cooking water. Mix the hot potatoes with half of your dressing so they absorb the flavors. After the potatoes have cooled, toss them with the remaining dressing.

Roasted Broccoli Panzanella Salad

DAIRY-FREE, NUT-FREE, EGG-FREE, VEGETARIAN, 5 INGREDIENTS

Panzanella is a traditional peasant salad from Tuscany made of chopped day-old bread and tomatoes. This salad can be dressed ahead of time and it won't wilt, so it's perfect for a picnic.

1 pound broccoli (about 3 medium stalks), trimmed, cut into 1-inch florets and ½-inch stem slices

3 tablespoons extra-virgin olive oil, divided

1 pint cherry or grape tomatoes (about 1½ cups)

1½ teaspoons honey, divided

3 cups cubed whole-grain crusty bread

1 tablespoon balsamic vinegar

½ teaspoon freshly ground black pepper

¼ teaspoon kosher or sea salt

Grated Parmesan cheese (or other hard cheese) and chopped fresh oregano leaves, for serving (optional)

Per Serving Calories: 226; Total Fat: 12g; Saturated Fat: 2g; Cholesterol: 0mg; Sodium: 287mg; Total Carbohydrates: 26g; Fiber: 6g; Protein: 7g

1. Place a large, rimmed baking sheet in the oven. Preheat the oven to 450°F with the pan inside.

2. Put the broccoli in a large bowl, and drizzle with 1 tablespoon of the oil. Toss to coat.

3. Carefully remove the hot baking sheet from the oven and spoon the broccoli onto it, leaving some oil in the bottom of the bowl. Add the tomatoes to the same bowl, and toss to coat with the leftover oil (don't add any more oil). Toss the tomatoes with 1 teaspoon of honey, and scrape them onto the baking sheet with the broccoli.

4. Roast for 15 minutes, stirring halfway through. Remove the sheet from the oven, and add the bread cubes. Roast for 3 more minutes. The broccoli is ready when it appears slightly charred on the tips and is tender-crisp when poked with a fork.

5. Spoon the vegetable mixture onto a serving plate or into a large, flat bowl.

6. In a small bowl, whisk the remaining 2 tablespoons of oil together with the vinegar, the remaining ½ teaspoon of honey, and the pepper and salt. Pour over the salad, and toss gently. Sprinkle with cheese and oregano, if desired, and serve.

Prep tip: Don't toss those broccoli stems! Peel or thinly slice away the tough skin, then cut into ½-inch slices. When roasted, the stems are actually sweeter than the florets.

Pastina Chicken Soup with Kale

NUT-FREE, EGG-FREE, ONE POT

SERVES

6

PREP
TIME

5

COOK
TIME

25

At every Christmas get-together, Deanna's nana would make her version of Italian Wedding Soup for the first course. It would have pastina (tiny pasta), mini meatballs, and dark green escarole. If you were at the kids' table, you got the "strained" version (meaning without greens) by request, which every grandkid requested. Since then, Deanna's taste buds have grown up to favor hearty leafy greens, but if you aren't a big fan of kale, you can swap in spinach or broccoli.

1 tablespoon
extra-virgin olive oil

2 garlic cloves, minced
(about 1 teaspoon)

3 cups packed chopped
kale (center ribs removed)

1 cup minced carrots
(about 2 carrots)

8 cups low-sodium or
no-salt-added chicken
(or vegetable) broth

¼ teaspoon kosher
or sea salt

¼ teaspoon freshly
ground black pepper

¾ cup (6 ounces)
uncooked acini de pepe
or pastina pasta

2 cups shredded cooked
chicken (about 12 ounces)

3 tablespoons grated
Parmesan cheese

1. In a large stockpot over medium heat, heat the oil. Add the garlic and cook for 30 seconds, stirring frequently. Add the kale and carrots and cook for 5 minutes, stirring occasionally.

2. Add the broth, salt, and pepper, and turn the heat to high. Bring the broth to a boil, and add the pasta. Lower the heat to medium and cook for 10 minutes, or until the pasta is cooked through, stirring every few minutes so the pasta doesn't stick to the bottom. Add the chicken, and cook for 2 more minutes to warm through.

3. Ladle the soup into six bowls, top each with ½ tablespoon of cheese, and serve.

Ingredient tip: You can swap out the pastina in this soup for other grains, like couscous, farro, wild rice, or barley. Follow the directions on the package to get an idea of how long the grain should cook in the broth.

Per Serving Calories: 187; Total Fat: 5g; Saturated Fat: 1g; Cholesterol: 39mg; Sodium: 219mg; Total Carbohydrates: 16g; Fiber: 1g; Protein: 15g

Mushroom-Barley Soup

SERVES

6

PREP TIME

5

COOK TIME

25

NUT-FREE, EGG-FREE, VEGETARIAN, ONE POT

Yes, you can whip up a hearty, stick-to-your ribs soup in less than 30 minutes—one that also happens to be vegetarian. The cooked barley helps fill you up while delivering a healthy serving of grains. Don't forget the Parmesan on top—it gives the soup a hit of salty, tangy goodness. And just like almost all homemade soups, this one tastes even better the next day.

2 tablespoons extra-virgin olive oil

1 cup chopped onion (about ½ medium onion)

1 cup chopped carrots (about 2 carrots)

5½ cups chopped mushrooms (about 12 ounces)

6 cups low-sodium or no-salt-added vegetable broth

1 cup uncooked pearled barley

¼ cup red wine

2 tablespoons tomato paste

4 sprigs fresh thyme or ½ teaspoon dried thyme

1 dried bay leaf

6 tablespoons grated Parmesan cheese

1. In a large stockpot over medium heat, heat the oil. Add the onion and carrots and cook for 5 minutes, stirring frequently. Turn up the heat to medium-high and add the mushrooms. Cook for 3 minutes, stirring frequently.

2. Add the broth, barley, wine, tomato paste, thyme, and bay leaf. Stir, cover the pot, and bring the soup to a boil. Once it's boiling, stir a few times, reduce the heat to medium-low, cover, and cook for another 12 to 15 minutes, until the barley is cooked through.

3. Remove the bay leaf and serve in soup bowls with 1 tablespoon of cheese sprinkled on top of each.

Ingredient tip: Tomato paste is a concentrated flavor bomb that instantly makes any dish more robust. The problem is you typically only need a few tablespoons per recipe, leaving a lot left over in the can. Solution: Spoon the remaining paste in 1-tablespoon amounts into an ice cube tray and freeze. Once frozen, pop the cubes into a freezer bag and store in the freezer until the next time you need tomato paste for a recipe.

Per Serving Calories: 236; Total Fat: 7g; Saturated Fat: 2g; Cholesterol: 5mg; Sodium: 231mg; Total Carbohydrates: 35g; Fiber: 7g; Protein: 8g

Easy Pasta Fagioli Soup

NUT-FREE, EGG-FREE, VEGETARIAN, ONE POT

SERVES

6

PREP TIME

5

COOK TIME

25

Pasta e fagioli—pronounced "pasta fazool" by us non-Italians—is a thick, comforting soup. Despite the fact that it's vegetarian, it's packed with protein and is very filling. Store any leftovers in the refrigerator and enjoy it over several days as the ingredients continue to grow richer in flavor.

2 tablespoons extra-virgin olive oil

½ cup chopped onion (about ¼ onion)

3 garlic cloves, minced (about 1½ teaspoons)

1 tablespoon minced fresh rosemary or 1 teaspoon dried rosemary

¼ teaspoon crushed red pepper

4 cups low-sodium or no-salt-added vegetable broth

2 (15.5-ounce) cans cannellini, great northern, or light kidney beans, undrained

1 (28-ounce) can low-sodium or no-salt-added crushed tomatoes

2 tablespoons tomato paste

8 ounces uncooked short pasta, such as ditalini, tubetti, or elbows

6 tablespoons grated Parmesan cheese (about 1½ ounces)

1. In a large stockpot over medium heat, heat the oil. Add the onion and cook for 4 minutes, stirring frequently. Add the garlic, rosemary, and crushed red pepper. Cook for 1 minute, stirring frequently. Add the broth, canned beans with their liquid, tomatoes, and tomato paste. Simmer for 5 minutes.

2. To thicken the soup, carefully transfer 2 cups to a blender. Purée, then stir it back into the pot.

3. Bring the soup to a boil over high heat. Mix in the pasta, and lower the heat to a simmer. Cook the pasta for the amount of time recommended on the box, stirring every few minutes to prevent the pasta from sticking to the pot. Taste the pasta to make sure it is cooked through (it could take a few more minutes than the recommended cooking time, since it's cooking with other ingredients).

4. Ladle the soup into bowls, top each with 1 tablespoon of grated cheese, and serve.

Ingredient tip: Deanna often adds whatever extra leafy greens she has in her refrigerator to this soup—like kale, spinach, or arugula, for an extra punch of nutrition and flavor. Add up to 3 cups total of the greens once the soup is cooked in step 4, then let them sit for 5 minutes in the hot soup to wilt.

Per Serving Calories: 382; Total Fat: 8g; Saturated Fat: 2g; Cholesterol: 5mg; Sodium: 620mg; Total Carbohydrates: 56g; Fiber: 9g; Protein: 15g

Roasted Carrot Soup with Parmesan Croutons

SERVES

4

PREP
TIME

10

COOK
TIME

20

NUT-FREE, EGG-FREE, VEGETARIAN

Roasting intensifies the sweetness of root vegetables like carrots, sweet potatoes, beets, and parsnips. It's what makes this gorgeous carrot soup go from good to sensational. But it can take up to 45 minutes of oven time before those veggies caramelize and are cooked through. Our shortcut is to place the sheet pan in the oven before adding finely sliced carrots, slashing the usual roasting time.

2 pounds carrots, unpeeled, cut into ½-inch slices (about 6 cups)

2 tablespoons extra-virgin olive oil, divided

1 cup chopped onion (about ½ medium onion)

2 cups low-sodium or no-salt-added vegetable (or chicken) broth

2½ cups water

1 teaspoon dried thyme

¼ teaspoon crushed red pepper

¼ teaspoon kosher or sea salt

4 thin slices whole-grain bread

1/3 cup freshly grated Parmesan cheese (about 1 ounce)

1. Place one oven rack about four inches below the broiler element. Place two large, rimmed baking sheets in the oven on any oven rack. Preheat the oven to 450°F.

2. In a large bowl, toss the carrots with 1 tablespoon of oil to coat. With oven mitts, carefully remove the baking sheets from the oven and evenly distribute the carrots on both sheets. Bake for 20 minutes, until the carrots are just fork tender, stirring once halfway through. The carrots will still be somewhat firm. Remove the carrots from the oven, and turn the oven to the high broil setting.

3. While the carrots are roasting, in a large stockpot over medium-high heat, heat 1 tablespoon of oil. Add the onion and cook for 5 minutes, stirring occasionally. Add the broth, water, thyme, crushed red pepper, and salt. Bring to a boil, cover, then remove the pan from the heat until the carrots have finished roasting.

4. Add the roasted carrots to the pot, and blend with an immersion blender (or use a regular blender—carefully pour in the hot soup in batches, then return the soup to the pot). Heat the soup for about 1 minute over medium-high heat, until warmed through.

5. Turn the oven to the high broil setting. Place the bread on the baking sheet. Sprinkle the cheese evenly across the slices of bread. Broil the bread 4 inches below the heating element for 1 to 2 minutes, or until the cheese melts, watching carefully to prevent burning.

6. Cut the bread into bite-size croutons. Divide the soup evenly among four bowls, top each with the Parmesan croutons, and serve.

Prep tip: Did you know that you can eat the skin of many vegetables that we typically peel? Not only do you save time and avoid waste by not peeling, but many of a plant's potent phytonutrients are found right below their skin. Keep the fiber-rich skins on carrots, cucumbers, eggplant, zucchini, potatoes, sweet potatoes, and beets.

Per Serving Calories: 272; Total Fat: 10g; Saturated Fat: 2g; Cholesterol: 5mg; Sodium: 520mg; Total Carbohydrates: 38g; Fiber: 8g; Protein: 10g

Paella Soup

DAIRY-FREE, NUT-FREE, GLUTEN-FREE, EGG-FREE, ONE POT

Paella is a Spanish rice dish that contains seafood and often spicy chorizo sausage—and it takes over an hour to make. This thick, quick-cook soup version takes half the time, using shrimp and instant brown rice. Saffron seasons traditional paella and gives it a beautiful yellow-orange color, but it can be expensive, so we use more budget-friendly, antioxidant-rich turmeric to get the same golden color.

1 cup frozen green peas

2 tablespoons
extra-virgin olive oil

1 cup chopped onion
(about ½ medium onion)

1½ cups coarsely
chopped red bell pepper
(about 1 large pepper)

1½ cups coarsely chopped
green bell pepper (about
1 large pepper)

2 garlic cloves, chopped
(about 1 teaspoon)

1 teaspoon ground turmeric

1 teaspoon dried thyme

2 teaspoons
smoked paprika

2½ cups uncooked
instant brown rice

2 cups low-sodium
or no-salt-added
chicken broth

2½ cups water

1 (28-ounce) can
low-sodium or no-salt-
added crushed tomatoes

1 pound fresh raw
medium shrimp (or
frozen raw shrimp
completely thawed),
shells and tails removed

1. Put the frozen peas on the counter to partially thaw as the soup is being prepared.

2. In a large stockpot over medium-high heat, heat the oil. Add the onion, red and green bell peppers, and garlic. Cook for 8 minutes, stirring occasionally. Add the turmeric, thyme, and smoked paprika, and cook for 2 minutes more, stirring often. Stir in the rice, broth, and water. Bring to a boil over high heat. Cover, reduce the heat to medium-low, and cook for 10 minutes.

3. Stir the peas, tomatoes, and shrimp into the soup. Cook for 4 to 6 minutes, until the shrimp is cooked, turning from gray to pink and white. The soup will be very thick, almost like stew, when ready to serve.

Ingredient tip: We love using frozen shrimp for the price and convenience, plus they're frozen right after harvesting, so they're often fresher than raw shrimp at the fish counter. To thaw, place them in a colander set in a bowl. Cover with plastic wrap and refrigerate overnight. For a faster thaw, put the frozen shrimp in a bowl of cold water and thaw for 20 minutes, changing the water halfway through the process.

Per Serving Calories: 342; Total Fat: 8g; Saturated Fat: 1g; Cholesterol: 148mg; Sodium: 253mg; Total Carbohydrates: 48g; Fiber: 5g; Protein: 24g

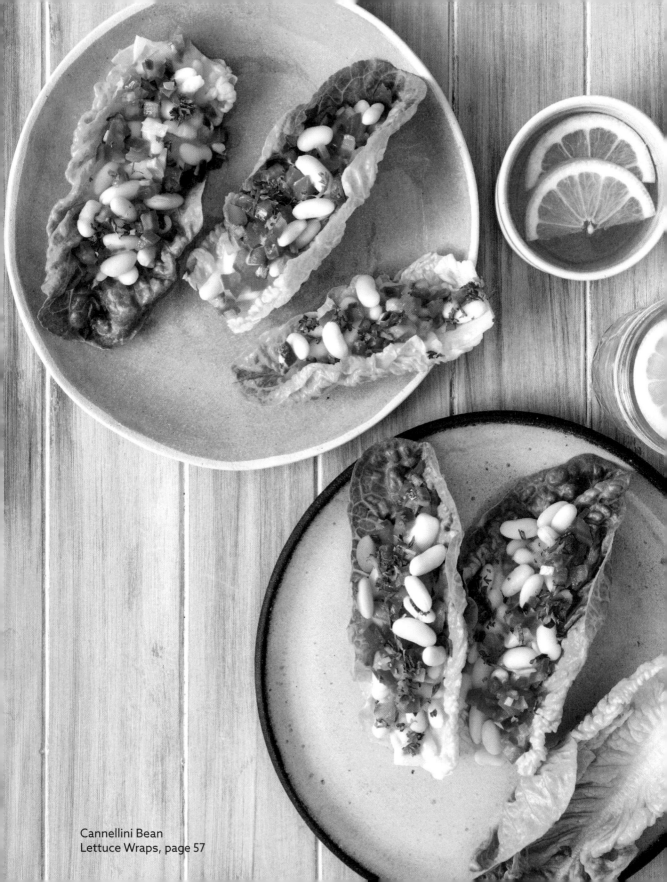

Cannellini Bean
Lettuce Wraps, page 57

FIVE

Beans, Rice, and Grains

EMBRACE the carbs! From Italian Baked Beans (page 56) to Brown Rice Pilaf with Golden Raisins (page 61), this chapter showcases the foundation of the Mediterranean Diet: rice, whole grains, and beans, which are loaded with B vitamins, fiber, protein, antioxidants, iron, and more. We use lots of fresh, easy-to-find herbs and super spices to transform these plant-based foods from basic to bravo. Also, these recipes are very adaptable—serve them as a side dish with one of our soups or meat dishes, or increase the portion size, add some leftover chicken or fish, and serve them as a main meal.

Italian Baked Beans

SERVES

6

PREP TIME

5

COOK TIME

15

This Mediterranean twist on baked beans features the delightful combination of honey, cinnamon, and homemade ketchup. The ketchup is so simple to make, you might even give up the store-bought bottle (it's that good)! Just turn off the heat at the end of step 1, and it's ready! Serve these beans as a side dish at a cookout, or pour them over your favorite bowl of grains.

2 teaspoons extra-virgin olive oil

½ cup minced onion (about ¼ onion)

1 (12-ounce) can low-sodium tomato paste

¼ cup red wine vinegar

2 tablespoons honey

¼ teaspoon ground cinnamon

½ cup water

2 (15-ounce) cans cannellini or great northern beans, undrained

Per Serving Calories: 236; Total Fat: 3g; Saturated Fat: 1g; Cholesterol: 0mg; Sodium: 440mg; Total Carbohydrates: 42g; Fiber: 11g; Protein: 10g

1. In a medium saucepan over medium heat, heat the oil. Add the onion and cook for 5 minutes, stirring frequently. Add the tomato paste, vinegar, honey, cinnamon, and water, and mix well. Turn the heat to low.

2. Drain and rinse one can of the beans in a colander and add to the saucepan. Pour the entire second can of beans (including the liquid) into the saucepan. Let it cook for 10 minutes, stirring occasionally, and serve.

Ingredient tip: Switch up this recipe by making new variations of the homemade ketchup. Instead of the cinnamon, try ¼ teaspoon of smoked paprika and 1 tablespoon of hot sauce. Or use ¼ teaspoon of dried oregano and 1 tablespoon of diced olives instead of the cinnamon.

Cannellini Bean Lettuce Wraps

GLUTEN-FREE, VEGAN, ONE POT

SERVES

4

PREP
TIME

10

COOK
TIME

10

Lettuce wraps are easy to make and extremely versatile as an appetizer or lunch—you can stuff them with anything from nutritious grain salads to savory seafood. Plus, they're a terrific option for those who need to follow a gluten-free lifestyle. For a Mediterranean spin, we spoon a warm, buttery bean filling onto crisp leaves of romaine lettuce and then slather on our Lemony Garlic Hummus (page 31).

1 tablespoon
extra-virgin olive oil

½ cup diced red onion
(about ¼ onion)

¾ cup chopped fresh
tomatoes (about
1 medium tomato)

¼ teaspoon freshly
ground black pepper

1 (15-ounce) can cannellini
or great northern beans,
drained and rinsed

¼ cup finely chopped
fresh curly parsley

½ cup Lemony Garlic
Hummus (page 31) or
½ cup prepared hummus

8 romaine lettuce leaves

Per Serving Calories: 211; Total
Fat: 8g; Saturated Fat: 1g; Choles-
terol: 0mg; Sodium: 368mg; Total
Carbohydrates: 28g; Fiber: 8g;
Protein: 10g

1. In a large skillet over medium heat, heat the oil. Add the onion and cook for 3 minutes, stirring occasionally. Add the tomatoes and pepper and cook for 3 more minutes, stirring occasionally. Add the beans and cook for 3 more minutes, stirring occasionally. Remove from the heat, and mix in the parsley.

2. Spread 1 tablespoon of hummus over each lettuce leaf. Evenly spread the warm bean mixture down the center of each leaf. Fold one side of the lettuce leaf over the filling lengthwise, then fold over the other side to make a wrap and serve.

Ingredient tip: Leafy romaine is our go-to choice for lettuce wraps because of its long leaves and sturdy yet pleasantly crisp, edible stems. Other options are green leaf, red leaf, Boston, or Bibb lettuces. You can also use heartier greens like kale, cabbage, Swiss chard, and collards; they just need to be parboiled or steamed before wrapping. Check out our Greek Stuffed Collard Greens (page 112) for tips on how to use these heartier greens as wraps.

Israeli Eggplant, Chickpea, and Mint Sauté

SERVES

6

PREP TIME

5

COOK TIME

20

If you don't really like eggplant, we encourage you to try this recipe, which turns that tough eggplant interior silky and luxurious. This vibrant sauté includes many ingredients found in the classic Middle Eastern dip baba ghanoush. Serve this as a vegetarian main or a side dish with some whole-grain crusty bread to soak up the tangy dressing.

Nonstick cooking spray

1 medium globe eggplant (about 1 pound), stem removed

1 tablespoon extra-virgin olive oil

2 tablespoons freshly squeezed lemon juice (from about 1 small lemon)

2 tablespoons balsamic vinegar

1 teaspoon ground cumin

¼ teaspoon kosher or sea salt

1 (15-ounce) can chickpeas, drained and rinsed

1 cup sliced sweet onion (about ½ medium Walla Walla or Vidalia onion)

¼ cup loosely packed chopped or torn mint leaves

1 tablespoon sesame seeds, toasted if desired

1 garlic clove, finely minced (about ½ teaspoon)

1. Place one oven rack about 4 inches below the broiler element. Turn the broiler to the highest setting to preheat. Spray a large, rimmed baking sheet with nonstick cooking spray.

2. On a cutting board, cut the eggplant lengthwise into four slabs (each piece should be about ½- to ⅝-inch thick). Place the eggplant slabs on the prepared baking sheet. Set aside.

3. In a small bowl, whisk together the oil, lemon juice, vinegar, cumin, and salt. Brush or drizzle 2 tablespoons of the lemon dressing over both sides of the eggplant slabs. Reserve the remaining dressing.

4. Broil the eggplant directly under the heating element for 4 minutes, flip them, then broil for another 4 minutes, until golden brown.

5. While the eggplant is broiling, in a serving bowl, combine the chickpeas, onion, mint, sesame seeds, and garlic. Add the reserved dressing, and gently mix to incorporate all the ingredients.

6. When the eggplant is done, using tongs, transfer the slabs from the baking sheet to a cooling rack and cool for 3 minutes. When slightly cooled, place the eggplant on a cutting board and slice each slab crosswise into ½-inch strips.

7. Add the eggplant to the serving bowl with the onion mixture. Gently toss everything together, and serve warm or at room temperature.

Prep tip: It usually takes about 30 minutes in the oven to turn the texture of eggplant creamy and soft. Here, we use a quick broiling method that makes that magic happen in only 8 minutes. Because the eggplant slabs have a greater surface area than a whole eggplant and the broiler gives off intense heat, the vegetable softens quickly.

Per Serving Calories: 159; Total Fat: 4g; Saturated Fat: 1g; Cholesterol: 0mg; Sodium: 247mg; Total Carbohydrates: 26g; Fiber: 7g; Protein: 6g

Mediterranean Lentils and Rice

NUT-FREE, GLUTEN-FREE, VEGAN, ONE POT

Lentils and rice are the Mediterranean equivalent of Latin American rice and beans. And because this recipe doesn't contain meat, fish, dairy, or eggs, it's an ideal choice to bring to picnics or cookouts where hot weather can compromise dishes sitting out in the sun too long.

2¼ cups low-sodium or no-salt-added vegetable broth

½ cup uncooked brown or green lentils

½ cup uncooked instant brown rice

½ cup diced carrots (about 1 carrot)

½ cup diced celery (about 1 stalk)

1 (2.25-ounce) can sliced olives, drained (about ½ cup)

¼ cup diced red onion (about ⅛ onion)

¼ cup chopped fresh curly-leaf parsley

1½ tablespoons extra-virgin olive oil

1 tablespoon freshly squeezed lemon juice (from about ½ small lemon)

1 garlic clove, minced (about ½ teaspoon)

¼ teaspoon kosher or sea salt

¼ teaspoon freshly ground black pepper

1. In a medium saucepan over high heat, bring the broth and lentils to a boil, cover, and lower the heat to medium-low. Cook for 8 minutes.

2. Raise the heat to medium, and stir in the rice. Cover the pot and cook the mixture for 15 minutes, or until the liquid is absorbed. Remove the pot from the heat and let it sit, covered, for 1 minute, then stir.

3. While the lentils and rice are cooking, mix together the carrots, celery, olives, onion, and parsley in a large serving bowl.

4. In a small bowl, whisk together the oil, lemon juice, garlic, salt, and pepper. Set aside.

5. When the lentils and rice are cooked, add them to the serving bowl. Pour the dressing on top, and mix everything together. Serve warm or cold, or store in a sealed container in the refrigerator for up to 7 days.

Ingredient tip: Confused over what type of fresh parsley to use in a dish? Think of flat-leaf or Italian parsley as spinach—it's more delicate and grassy tasting—while curly-leaf parsley is more like kale—hearty, with a coarser texture and touch of bitter flavor. Typically, flat-leaf is used in Italian dishes with pasta, chicken, and vegetables, and curly parsley is a staple in Greek and Middle Eastern fare, like chopped salads such as tabbouleh.

Per Serving Calories: 230; Total Fat: 8g; Saturated Fat: 1g; Cholesterol: 0mg; Sodium: 359mg; Total Carbohydrates: 34g; Fiber: 6g; Protein: 8g

Brown Rice Pilaf with Golden Raisins

GLUTEN-FREE, VEGAN, ONE POT

This Moroccan-inspired dish makes a super-flavorful side for a protein like chicken or fish. Or add chickpeas, and this becomes a vegan main dish. Serena also likes to warm up the leftovers, top it with Greek yogurt, and eat it for breakfast as an energizing way to start the day.

1 tablespoon
extra-virgin olive oil

1 cup chopped onion
(about ½ medium onion)

½ cup shredded carrot
(about 1 medium carrot)

1 teaspoon ground cumin

½ teaspoon ground
cinnamon

2 cups instant brown rice

1¾ cups 100% orange juice

¼ cup water

1 cup golden raisins

½ cup shelled pistachios

Chopped fresh
chives (optional)

1. In a medium saucepan over medium-high heat, heat the oil. Add the onion and cook for 5 minutes, stirring frequently. Add the carrot, cumin, and cinnamon, and cook for 1 minute, stirring frequently. Stir in the rice, orange juice, and water. Bring to a boil, cover, then lower the heat to medium-low. Simmer for 7 minutes, or until the rice is cooked through and the liquid is absorbed.

2. Stir in the raisins, pistachios, and chives (if using) and serve.

Prep tip: To bump up the nutrition and flavor of whole grains, cook them in low-sodium chicken or vegetable broth, coconut water, or orange juice, as we do here. This method is especially beneficial for whole grains with a bit of a bitter edge—like quinoa or sorghum—as cooking in a flavored liquid mellows their bite. Substitute these liquids for most or all of the water called for in the cooking directions on the grain package.

Per Serving Calories: 320;
Total Fat: 7g; Saturated Fat: 0g;
Cholesterol: 0mg; Sodium: 37mg;
Total Carbohydrates: 61g;
Fiber: 5g; Protein: 6g

Lebanese Rice and Broken Noodles with Cabbage

SERVES

6

PREP
TIME

5

COOK
TIME

25

NUT-FREE, VEGAN, ONE POT

Variations on rice and broken noodles are considered comfort food in many cultures. Traditionally, this simple dish is mainly made up of grain-based carbohydrates and a few aromatics, like onion, garlic, and occasionally herbs. Here, Serena adds her favorite vegetable, cabbage, which melts down into a mellow-tasting, pasta-like texture and contributes some important plant-based nutrients.

1 tablespoon
extra-virgin olive oil

1 cup (about 3 ounces)
uncooked vermicelli or
thin spaghetti, broken
into 1- to 1½-inch pieces

3 cups shredded cabbage
(about half a 14-ounce
package of coleslaw
mix or half a small
head of cabbage)

3 cups low-sodium
or no-salt-added
vegetable broth

½ cup water

1 cup instant brown rice

2 garlic cloves

¼ teaspoon kosher
or sea salt

1/8 to ¼ teaspoon
crushed red pepper

½ cup loosely packed,
coarsely chopped cilantro

Fresh lemon slices, for
serving (optional)

1. In a large saucepan over medium-high heat, heat the oil. Add the pasta and cook for 3 minutes to toast, stirring often. Add the cabbage and cook for 4 minutes, stirring often. Add the broth, water, rice, garlic, salt, and crushed red pepper, and bring to a boil over high heat. Stir, cover, and reduce the heat to medium-low. Simmer for 10 minutes.

2. Remove the pan from the heat, but do not lift the lid. Let sit for 5 minutes. Fish out the garlic cloves, mash them with a fork, then stir the garlic back into the rice. Stir in the cilantro. Serve with the lemon slices (if using).

Ingredient tip: Ever wondered what to do with a leftover half head of cabbage or half a package of coleslaw mix? We love to cook it in a tablespoon of olive oil with chopped onion, then add it to canned soup, scrambled eggs, tacos, or even leftover rice for stir-fried rice.

Per Serving Calories: 259; Total Fat:4g; Saturated Fat: 1g; Cholesterol: 0mg; Sodium: 123mg; Total Carbohydrates: 49g; Fiber: 3g; Protein: 7g

Lemon Farro Bowl with Avocado

NUT-FREE, VEGAN, ONE POT

SERVES

6

PREP TIME

5

COOK TIME

25

Farro is an ancient strain of wheat that is popular in Italy. Luckily, this chewy, nutty grain is now widely available in the United States. You'll find it in the rice and grain aisle of most supermarkets. We use pearled farro here for its quicker cooking time. Pearled farro is not a whole grain but is rich in protein, fiber, and iron. Serve this as a side dish or even as a breakfast entrée, dividing the farro among four bowls and topping each with a cooked egg for more protein power.

1 tablespoon plus
2 teaspoons extra-virgin
olive oil, divided

1 cup chopped onion
(about ½ medium onion)

2 garlic cloves, minced
(about 1 teaspoon)

1 carrot, shredded
(about 1 cup)

2 cups low-sodium
or no-salt-added
vegetable broth

1 cup (6 ounces) uncooked
pearled or 10-minute farro

2 avocados, peeled,
pitted, and sliced

1 small lemon

¼ teaspoon kosher
or sea salt

1. In a medium saucepan over medium-high heat, heat 1 tablespoon of oil. Add the onion and cook for 5 minutes, stirring occasionally. Add the garlic and carrot and cook for 1 minute, stirring frequently. Add the broth and farro, and bring to a boil over high heat. Lower the heat to medium-low, cover, and simmer for about 20 minutes or until the farro is plump and slightly chewy (al dente).

2. Pour the farro into a serving bowl, and add the avocado slices. Using a Microplane or citrus zester, zest the peel of the lemon directly into the bowl of farro. Halve the lemon, and squeeze the juice out of both halves using a citrus juicer or your hands. Drizzle the remaining 2 teaspoons of oil over the bowl, and sprinkle with salt. Gently mix all the ingredients and serve.

Ingredient tip: Have you noticed we add lemon juice or vinegar to many of our recipes? If you've ever made a dish, tasted it, and thought something was missing, that something might be acid. Acidic ingredients like citrus juices and vinegars bring sparkle to dishes and give them an additional layer of flavor beyond just adding more salt.

Per Serving Calories: 279;
Total Fat: 14g; Saturated Fat:
2g; Cholesterol: 0mg; Sodium:
118mg; Total Carbohydrates: 36g;
Fiber: 9g; Protein: 7g

Barley Risotto with Parmesan

NUT-FREE, EGG-FREE, VEGETARIAN, 5 INGREDIENTS

SERVES

6

PREP
TIME

5

COOK
TIME

25

If you love risotto, the classic Italian dish made with creamy arborio rice, you'll love this updated version. This dish is made with barley instead of rice but uses the traditional risotto method of adding warm stock slowly so the grains cook up creamy. To make this a main dish to serve four, add a few cooked eggs on top.

4 cups low-sodium or no-salt-added vegetable broth

1 tablespoon extra-virgin olive oil

1 cup chopped yellow onion (about ½ medium onion)

2 cups uncooked pearl barley

½ cup dry white wine

1 cup freshly grated Parmesan cheese (about 4 ounces), divided

¼ teaspoon kosher or sea salt

¼ teaspoon freshly ground black pepper

Fresh chopped chives and lemon wedges, for serving (optional)

Per Serving Calories: 346; Total Fat: 7g; Saturated Fat: 3g; Cholesterol: 13mg; Sodium: 319mg; Total Carbohydrates: 56g; Fiber: 11g; Protein: 14g

1. Pour the broth into a medium saucepan and bring to a simmer.

2. In a large stockpot over medium-high heat, heat the oil. Add the onion and cook for 8 minutes, stirring occasionally. Add the barley and cook for 2 minutes, stirring until the barley is toasted. Pour in the wine and cook for about 1 minute, or until most of the liquid evaporates. Add 1 cup of warm broth to the pot and cook, stirring, for about 2 minutes, or until most of the liquid is absorbed. Add the remaining broth 1 cup at a time, cooking until each cup is absorbed (about 2 minutes each time) before adding the next. The last addition of broth will take a bit longer to absorb, about 4 minutes.

3. Remove the pot from the heat, and stir in ½ cup of cheese, and the salt and pepper. Serve with the remaining cheese on the side, along with the chives and lemon wedges (if using).

Ingredient tip: Pearled (quick) barley is not a whole grain, but it is high in protein and fiber and cooks in only 10 minutes, while whole-grain barley takes over an hour to cook. You may also find a new variety: whole hull-less barley, which takes about 40 minutes to cook.

Garlic-Asparagus Israeli Couscous

NUT-FREE, EGG-FREE, VEGETARIAN, 5 INGREDIENTS

SERVES

6

PREP TIME

5

COOK TIME

25

At the first hint of spring, look for asparagus at the store or the farmers' market and make this couscous dish. Israeli couscous is made from wheat flour and semolina and shaped like little pearls. The whole-wheat version is harder to find, but buy it if you see it at your store or online. You can also swap quinoa, farro, or brown rice for the couscous, cooking your grain of choice according to the package directions.

1 cup garlic-and-herb goat cheese (about 4 ounces)

1½ pounds asparagus spears, ends trimmed and stalks chopped into 1-inch pieces (about 2¾ to 3 cups chopped)

1 tablespoon extra-virgin olive oil

1 garlic clove, minced (about ½ teaspoon)

¼ teaspoon freshly ground black pepper

1¾ cups water

1 (8-ounce) box uncooked whole-wheat or regular Israeli couscous (about 1⅓ cups)

¼ teaspoon kosher or sea salt

Per Serving Calories: 263; Total Fat: 9g; Saturated Fat: 4g; Cholesterol: 15mg; Sodium: 162mg; Total Carbohydrates: 36g; Fiber: 3g; Protein: 11g

1. Preheat the oven to 425°F. Put the goat cheese on the counter to bring to room temperature.

2. In a large bowl, mix together the asparagus, oil, garlic, and pepper. Spread the asparagus on a large, rimmed baking sheet and roast for 10 minutes, stirring a few times. Remove the pan from the oven, and spoon the asparagus into a large serving bowl.

3. While the asparagus is roasting, in a medium saucepan, bring the water to a boil. Add the couscous and salt. Reduce the heat to medium-low, cover, and cook for 12 minutes, or until the water is absorbed.

4. Pour the hot couscous into the bowl with the asparagus. Add the goat cheese, mix thoroughly until completely melted, and serve.

Prep tip: Goat cheese melts into an instant creamy sauce when mixed with hot grains, as in this recipe. Ricotta cheese is an alternative here, along with adding in some fresh chopped herbs such as rosemary, basil, and/or oregano.

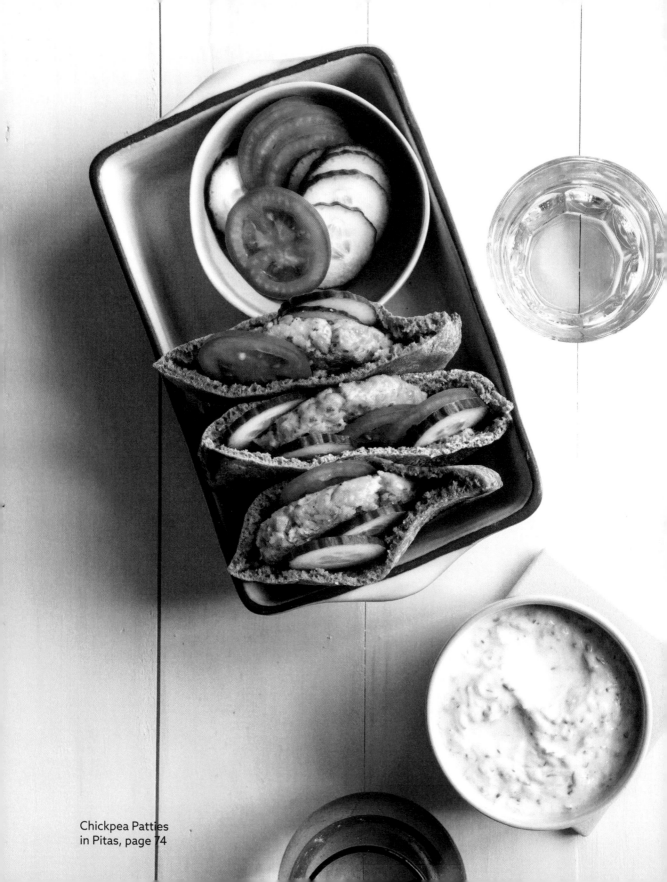

Chickpea Patties
in Pitas, page 74

SIX

Sandwiches and Wraps

GET out of your lunchtime rut with crave-worthy sandwiches and wraps. We've added some Mediterranean flair to many of the classics, like mixing olives into tuna salad and wrapping up chicken Parmesan in whole-wheat flatbread. Best of all, you can make several of these super sammies in 15 minutes or less, including Deanna's favorite recipe in this chapter, Prosciutto-Lettuce-Tomato-Avocado Sandwiches (page 68), a delectable Italian twist on the traditional BLT.

Prosciutto-Lettuce-Tomato-Avocado Sandwiches

SERVES

4

PREP
TIME

10

DAIRY-FREE, NUT-FREE, EGG-FREE, 5 INGREDIENTS, HALF THE TIME

We're upgrading your usual BLT with our irresistible PLTA! It has only five ingredients, but there's something magical about the combination of buttery avocado smeared on toasted bread and layered with crispy lettuce, juicy tomato, and thin slices of prosciutto.

8 slices whole-grain or whole-wheat bread

1 ripe avocado, halved and pitted

¼ teaspoon freshly ground black pepper

¼ teaspoon kosher or sea salt

4 romaine lettuce leaves, torn into 8 pieces total

1 large, ripe tomato, sliced into 8 rounds

2 ounces prosciutto, cut into 8 thin slices

Per Serving Calories: 240; Total Fat: 9g; Saturated Fat: 2g; Cholesterol: 8mg; Sodium: 558mg; Total Carbohydrates: 29g; Fiber: 7g; Protein: 12g

1. Toast the bread and place on a large platter.

2. Scoop the avocado flesh out of the skin into a small bowl. Add the pepper and salt. Using a fork or a whisk, gently mash the avocado until it resembles a creamy spread. Spread the avocado mash over all 8 pieces of toast.

3. To make one sandwich, take one slice of avocado toast, and top it with a lettuce leaf, tomato slice, and prosciutto slice. Top with another slice each of lettuce, tomato, and prosciutto, then cover with a second piece of avocado toast (avocado-side down on the prosciutto). Repeat with the remaining ingredients to make three more sandwiches and serve.

Prep tip: Place the avocado standing up on your cutting board (with the stem end up). Slice the fruit down and in half, maneuvering your knife around the pit. Then simply twist the two sides and pull them apart. Scoop the pit out with a spoon.

Italian Tuna Sandwiches

This zesty sandwich filling brings to mind a leisurely lunch with a glass of wine while lounging at a sunny Italian seaside café. Bright lemon, spicy black pepper, and anise-flavored fresh fennel come together to make a simple tuna sandwich something special. Serve sandwich-style on crusty whole-grain bread or try the tuna atop salad greens.

3 tablespoons freshly squeezed lemon juice (from 1 medium lemon)

2 tablespoons extra-virgin olive oil

1 garlic clove, minced (about ½ teaspoon)

½ teaspoon freshly ground black pepper

2 (5-ounce) cans tuna, drained

1 (2.25-ounce) can sliced olives, any green or black variety (about ½ cup)

½ cup chopped fresh fennel, including fronds, or celery (about 1 stalk), including leaves

8 slices whole-grain crusty bread

1. In a medium bowl, whisk to combine the lemon juice, oil, garlic, and pepper. Add the tuna, olives, and fennel. Using a fork, separate the tuna into chunks and stir to combine all the ingredients.

2. Divide the tuna salad equally among 4 slices of bread. Top each with the remaining bread slices. Let the sandwiches sit for at least 5 minutes so the zesty filling can soak into the bread before serving.

Ingredient tip: Comparing canned tunas, we think the richer, better-tasting option is tuna packed in olive oil, which has only about 40 calories more per serving compared to water-packed tuna. We encourage you to do a taste test to see the flavor difference (if you aren't already a convert).

Per Serving Calories: 347; Total Fat: 17g; Saturated Fat: 3g; Cholesterol: 22mg; Sodium: 487mg; Total Carbohydrates: 27g; Fiber: 5g; Protein: 25g

Margherita Open-Face Sandwiches

NUT-FREE, EGG-FREE, VEGETARIAN, HALF THE TIME, ONE POT

SERVES

4

PREP TIME

10

COOK TIME

5

Traditional Margherita pizza features the colors of the Italian flag, with its vibrant tomato sauce, fresh mozzarella, and bright basil leaf toppings. Here's our shortcut sandwich version of the classic, made in minutes under your broiler. See the prep tip to avoid making green, white, red, and black (as in burnt) Margherita sandwiches.

2 (6- to 7-inch) whole-wheat submarine or hoagie rolls, sliced open horizontally

1 tablespoon extra-virgin olive oil

1 garlic clove, halved

1 large ripe tomato, cut into 8 slices

¼ teaspoon dried oregano

1 cup fresh mozzarella (about 4 ounces), patted dry and sliced

¼ cup lightly packed fresh basil leaves, torn into small pieces

¼ teaspoon freshly ground black pepper

1. Preheat the broiler to high with the rack 4 inches under the heating element.

2. Place the sliced bread on a large, rimmed baking sheet. Place under the broiler for 1 minute, until the bread is just lightly toasted. Remove from the oven.

3. Brush each piece of the toasted bread with the oil, and rub a garlic half over each piece.

4. Place the toasted bread back on the baking sheet. Evenly distribute the tomato slices on each piece, sprinkle with the oregano, and layer the cheese on top.

5. Place the baking sheet under the broiler. Set the timer for 1½ minutes, but check after 1 minute. When the cheese is melted and the edges are just starting to get dark brown, remove the sandwiches from the oven (this can take anywhere from 1½ to 2 minutes).

6. Top each sandwich with the fresh basil and pepper.

Prep tip: When using your broiler, follow these tips to avoid burnt toast and overly blackened foods: 1) Make sure your broiler is preheated. 2) Know where your rack is—the closer to the heat, the quicker the burn. 3) Set a timer and stay near the oven to check the progress. Sometimes it's a mere 10-second difference between your open-face sandwich being perfectly melted and setting off the smoke alarm. (Deanna speaks from many years of experience of losing out to her broiler.)

Per Serving Calories 297; Total Fat: 11g; Saturated Fat: 5g; Cholesterol: 22mg; Sodium: 450mg; Total Carbohydrates: 38g; Fiber: 4g; Protein: 12g

Roasted Veggie Panini

NUT-FREE, EGG-FREE, VEGETARIAN

Take your grilled cheese sandwich to the next level by loading it with savory roasted veggies. This gooey, cheesy panini is stuffed with broccoli, zucchini, onions, and peppers, but you can sub just about any veggie you'd like (we love it with tomatoes, mushrooms, and broccoli rabe, too).

2 tablespoons extra-virgin olive oil, divided

1½ cups diced broccoli (about 1 large stalk)

1 cup diced zucchini (about ½ large zucchini)

¼ cup diced onion (about 1/8 onion)

¼ teaspoon dried oregano

1/8 teaspoon freshly ground black pepper

1/8 teaspoon kosher or sea salt

Nonstick cooking spray

1 (12-ounce) jar roasted red peppers, drained and finely chopped

2 tablespoons grated Parmesan or Asiago cheese

1 cup fresh mozzarella (about 4 ounces), sliced

1 (2-foot-long) whole-grain Italian loaf, cut into 4 equal lengths

1. Place a large, rimmed baking sheet in the oven. Preheat the oven to 450°F with the pan inside.

2. In a large bowl, mix together 1 tablespoon of oil with the broccoli, zucchini, onion, oregano, pepper, and salt.

3. Remove the baking sheet from the oven, and carefully coat the pan with nonstick cooking spray. Spread the vegetable mixture on the pan and roast for 5 minutes, stirring once halfway through cooking.

4. Remove the pan from the oven. Add the red peppers and Parmesan cheese to the vegetables on the baking sheet and mix together.

5. In your panini maker, grill pan, or large skillet over medium-high heat, heat the remaining table-spoon of oil.

6. Cut open each section of bread horizontally, but don't cut all the way through. Fill each with the vegetable mix (about ½ cup), and layer 1 ounce of sliced mozzarella cheese on top. Close the sandwiches, and place two of them on the panini press, pan, or skillet. If you're using a panini press, close it and grill for 3 to 5 minutes, or until the crust is golden and the cheese has melted. For a pan or skillet, place a heavy object on top (see tip), and grill for 2½ minutes. Flip the sandwiches and grill for another 2½ minutes.

7. Repeat the grilling process with the remaining two sandwiches.

Prep tip: You don't need a fancy panini maker to enjoy this sandwich. Deanna makes paninis on her grill pan with her tea kettle resting on top as the weight. Other options to press your panini include using another skillet, a large plate, a pot lid, or even a brick wrapped in foil placed on top of the sandwich as it cooks.

Per Serving Calories: 352; Total Fat: 15g; Saturated Fat: 5g; Cholesterol: 12mg; Sodium: 658mg; Total Carbohydrates: 45g; Fiber: 2g; Protein: 16g

Chickpea Patties in Pitas

SERVES

4

PREP TIME

10

COOK TIME

15

This easy weeknight meal is our quick twist on the beloved Mediterranean street food falafel. Serena first tasted these crunchy chickpea fritters wrapped in warm pita bread from a street vendor in Greece years ago. Here, we use our homemade hummus as a way to easily bind the patties while also adding robust flavor. Creamy tzatziki, a refreshing cucumber yogurt sauce, ties together this simple yet memorable sandwich.

1 (15-ounce) can chickpeas, drained and rinsed

½ cup Lemony Garlic Hummus (page 31) or ½ cup prepared hummus

½ cup whole-wheat panko bread crumbs

1 large egg

2 teaspoons dried oregano

¼ teaspoon freshly ground black pepper

1 tablespoon extra-virgin olive oil

1 cucumber, unpeeled (or peeled if desired), cut in half lengthwise

1 (6-ounce) container 2% plain Greek yogurt

1 garlic clove, minced (about ½ teaspoon)

2 whole-wheat pita breads, cut in half

1 medium tomato, cut into 4 thick slices

1. In a large bowl, mash the chickpeas with a potato masher or fork until coarsely smashed (they should still be somewhat chunky). Add the hummus, bread crumbs, egg, oregano, and pepper. Stir well to combine. With your hands, form the mixture into 4 (½-cup-size) patties. Press each patty flat to about ¾ inch thick and put on a plate.

2. In a large skillet over medium-high heat, heat the oil until very hot, about 3 minutes. Cook the patties for 5 minutes, then flip with a spatula. Cook for an additional 5 minutes.

3. While the patties are cooking, shred half of the cucumber with a box grater or finely chop with a knife. In a small bowl, stir together the shredded cucumber, yogurt, and garlic to make the tzatziki sauce. Slice the remaining half of the cucumber into ¼-inch-thick slices and set aside.

4. Toast the pita breads. To assemble the sandwiches, lay the pita halves on a work surface. Into each pita, place a few slices of cucumber, a chickpea patty, and a tomato slice, then drizzle the sandwich with the tzatziki sauce and serve.

Ingredient tip: Bottled or jarred dried herbs and ground spices can lose their potent flavor after just 6 months, even if stored properly away from heat and light. To revive dried herbs, crumble them between your fingertips as you drop into a dish. To revive older spices, place the amount needed in a dry pan and cook over medium heat, stirring constantly, for about 1 minute to toast.

Per Serving Calories: 375; Total Fat: 12g; Saturated Fat: 2g; Cholesterol: 49mg; Sodium: 632mg; Total Carbohydrates: 53g; Fiber: 10g; Protein: 17g

Greek Salad Wraps

NUT-FREE, EGG-FREE, VEGETARIAN

SERVES

4

PREP TIME

15

This wrap features all the best ingredients of a Greek salad. We also like to use a decent-size portion of fresh herbs—here it's sweet, vibrant mint—to complement or even replace the typical salad greens. But feel free to also mix in some spinach, arugula, or another favorite leafy green to get in another serving of veggies.

1½ cups seedless cucumber, peeled and chopped (about 1 large cucumber)

1 cup chopped tomato (about 1 large tomato)

½ cup finely chopped fresh mint

1 (2.25-ounce) can sliced black olives (about ½ cup), drained

¼ cup diced red onion (about ¼ onion)

2 tablespoons extra-virgin olive oil

1 tablespoon red wine vinegar

¼ teaspoon freshly ground black pepper

¼ teaspoon kosher or sea salt

½ cup crumbled goat cheese (about 2 ounces)

4 whole-wheat flatbread wraps or soft whole-wheat tortillas

1. In a large bowl, mix together the cucumber, tomato, mint, olives, and onion until well combined.

2. In a small bowl, whisk together the oil, vinegar, pepper, and salt. Drizzle the dressing over the salad, and mix gently.

3. With a knife, spread the goat cheese evenly over the four wraps. Spoon a quarter of the salad filling down the middle of each wrap.

4. Fold up each wrap: Start by folding up the bottom, then fold one side over and fold the other side over the top. Repeat with the remaining wraps and serve.

Prep tip: Raw red onions add a sharp, tangy bite to many dishes, but we all know they don't leave us with the freshest breath. To mellow out their powerful flavor, put your thinly sliced onions in a bowl of ice water (make sure the water is covering the onions). Let them sit for about 15 minutes before draining.

Per Serving Calories: 262; Total Fat: 15g; Saturated Fat: 5g; Cholesterol: 15mg; Sodium: 529mg; Total Carbohydrates: 23g; Fiber: 4g; Protein: 7g

Dill Salmon Salad Wraps

DAIRY-FREE, NUT-FREE, EGG-FREE, HALF THE TIME

SERVES

6

PREP
TIME

10

COOK
TIME

10

True to the Mediterranean style of preparing food, this delicious sandwich is simple to make but relies on high-quality ingredients—like extra-virgin olive oil and aged balsamic vinegar, which is more syrupy than regular balsamic. If you want to skip the bread, enjoy this salad over a bed of arugula or brown rice.

1 pound salmon filet, cooked and flaked, or 3 (5-ounce) cans salmon

½ cup diced carrots (about 1 carrot)

½ cup diced celery (about 1 celery stalk)

3 tablespoons chopped fresh dill

3 tablespoons diced red onion (a little less than 1/8 onion)

2 tablespoons capers

1½ tablespoons extra-virgin olive oil

1 tablespoon aged balsamic vinegar

½ teaspoon freshly ground black pepper

¼ teaspoon kosher or sea salt

4 whole-wheat flatbread wraps or soft whole-wheat tortillas

1. In a large bowl, mix together the salmon, carrots, celery, dill, red onion, capers, oil, vinegar, pepper, and salt.

2. Divide the salmon salad among the flatbreads. Fold up the bottom of the flatbread, then roll up the wrap and serve.

Prep tip: If you are cooking the salmon instead of using canned, place a rack about 4 inches under your oven broiler and turn the broiler on high. Cook for about 10 minutes, or until the salmon flakes easily. Cool slightly before mixing the salmon with the remaining sandwich ingredients.

Per Serving Calories: 336; Total Fat: 16g; Saturated Fat: 2g; Cholesterol: 67mg; Sodium: 628mg; Total Carbohydrates: 23g; Fiber: 5g; Protein: 32g

Chicken Parmesan Wraps

When Serena first tested this recipe, her kids didn't want the chicken sliced into strips. Instead, they wrapped up the entire chicken breast in a green spinach wrap "like a Christmas present." They thought it was easier (and more fun!) to eat the chicken breast whole. Either way—with the chicken whole or sliced—everyone will love this saucy, melty, cheesy, and a bit messy Italian classic, served up sandwich style.

SERVES

6

PREP TIME

10

COOK TIME

20

Nonstick cooking spray

1 pound boneless, skinless chicken breasts

1 large egg

¼ cup buttermilk

⅔ cup whole-wheat panko or whole-wheat bread crumbs

½ cup grated Parmesan cheese (about 1½ ounces)

¾ teaspoon garlic powder, divided

1 cup canned low-sodium or no-salt-added crushed tomatoes

1 teaspoon dried oregano

6 (8-inch) whole-wheat tortillas, or whole-grain spinach wraps

1 cup fresh mozzarella cheese (about 4 ounces), sliced

1½ cups loosely packed fresh flat-leaf (Italian) parsley, chopped

1. Preheat the oven to 425°F. Line a large, rimmed baking sheet with aluminum foil. Place a wire rack on the aluminum foil, and spray the rack with nonstick cooking spray. Set aside.

2. Put the chicken breasts in a large, zip top plastic bag. With a rolling pin or meat mallet, pound the chicken so it is evenly flattened, about ¼ inch thick. Slice the chicken into six portions. (It's fine if you have to place 2 smaller pieces together to form six equal portions.)

3. In a wide, shallow bowl, whisk together the egg and buttermilk. In another wide, shallow bowl, mix together the panko crumbs, Parmesan cheese, and ½ teaspoon of garlic powder. Dip each chicken breast portion into the egg mixture and then into the Parmesan crumb mixture, pressing the crumbs into the chicken so they stick. Place the chicken on the prepared wire rack.

4. Bake the chicken for 15 to 18 minutes, or until the internal temperature of the chicken reads 165°F on a meat thermometer and any juices run clear. Transfer the chicken to a cutting board, and slice each portion diagonally into ½-inch pieces.

5. In a small, microwave-safe bowl, mix together the tomatoes, oregano, and the remaining ¼ teaspoon of garlic powder. Cover the bowl with a paper towel and microwave for about 1 minute on high, until very hot. Set aside.

6. Wrap the tortillas in a damp paper towel or dishcloth and microwave for 30 to 45 seconds on high, until warmed.

7. To assemble the wraps, divide the chicken slices evenly among the six tortillas and top with the cheese. Spread 1 tablespoon of the warm tomato sauce over the cheese on each tortilla, and top each with about ¼ cup of parsley. To wrap each tortilla, fold up the bottom of the tortilla, then fold one side over and fold the other side over the top. Serve the wraps immediately, with the remaining sauce for dipping.

Ingredient tip: In many Mediterranean countries, parsley and other fresh herbs are used more like salad rather than just a colorful garnish. Try adding herbs by the cupful to your salads, grain dishes, and wraps as a great way to use them up instead of seeing them become food waste.

Per Serving Calories: 373; Total Fat: 10g; Saturated Fat: 4g; Cholesterol: 95mg; Sodium: 591mg; Total Carbohydrates: 33g; Fiber: 8g; Protein: 30g

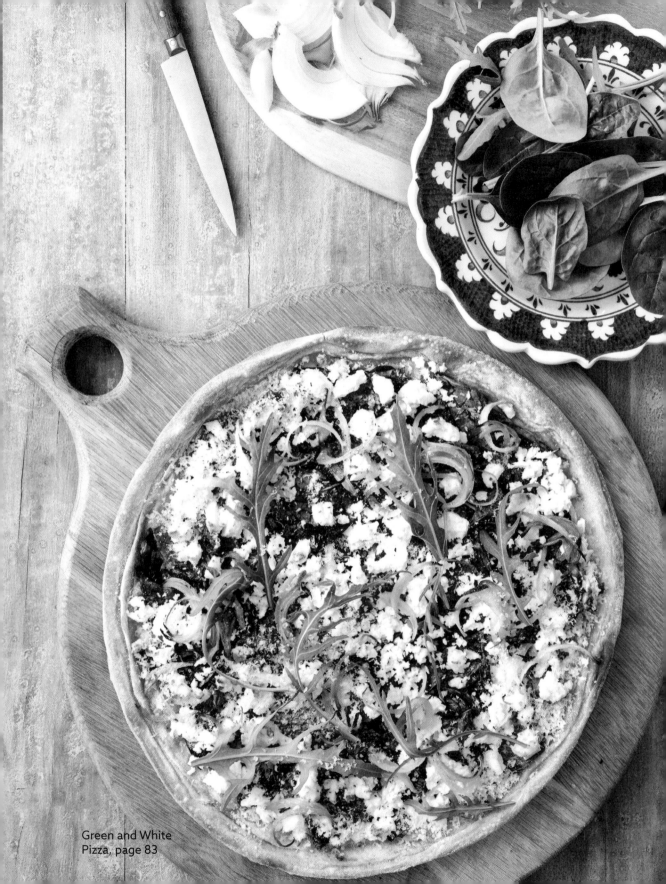

Green and White
Pizza, page 83

SEVEN

Pizza and Pasta

THIS is perhaps our most comfort food–filled collection in the book, where we share eight favorite mouthwatering, nutrient-packed pasta dishes and pizza pies. Pasta and pizza may have gotten a bad rap in recent years due to the rising popularity of low-carb diets. But we say, do what they do in Italy, and keep on enjoying the classics with some guidelines in mind: Keep portions reasonable, load on the veggie toppings or cook them into the sauce, then pair with lean proteins like fish, seafood, and beans.

Roasted Tomato Pita Pizzas

SERVES

6

PREP TIME

10

COOK TIME

20

If you like traditional tomato bruschetta topping, you'll love these easy-to-make pita pizzas. The roasted tomato sauce is super versatile (see the ingredient tip). And while the shortcut pizzas are delicious as is, feel free to pile on more Mediterranean-style toppings, from mushrooms to goat cheese to shrimp.

2 pints grape tomatoes (about 3 cups), halved

1 tablespoon extra-virgin olive oil

2 garlic cloves, minced (about 1 teaspoon)

1 teaspoon chopped fresh thyme leaves (from about 6 sprigs)

¼ teaspoon freshly ground black pepper

¼ teaspoon kosher or sea salt

¾ cup shredded Parmesan cheese (about 3 ounces)

6 whole-wheat pita breads

Per Serving Calories: 259; Total Fat: 7g; Saturated Fat: 3g; Cholesterol: 10mg; Sodium: 555mg; Total Carbohydrates: 40g; Fiber: 6g; Protein: 12g

1. Preheat the oven to 425°F.

2. In a baking pan, mix together the tomatoes, oil, garlic, thyme, pepper, and salt. Roast for 10 minutes. Pull out the rack, stir the tomatoes with a spatula or wooden spoon while still in the oven, and mash down the softened tomatoes to release more of their liquid. Roast for an additional 10 minutes.

3. While the tomatoes are roasting, sprinkle 2 tablespoons of cheese over each pita bread. Place the pitas on a large, rimmed baking sheet and toast in the oven for the last 5 minutes of the tomato cooking time.

4. Remove the tomato sauce and pita bread from the oven. Stir the tomatoes, spoon about ⅓ cup of sauce over each pita bread, and serve.

Ingredient tip: Deanna makes this roasted tomato topping almost every week (usually adding in ½ teaspoon of smoked paprika). It's versatile enough to use as a chunky sauce (as in our Salmon Skillet Supper on page 101); as a flavorful spread over chicken, fish, or seafood; or as a topper for burgers. She prefers using grape tomatoes or larger plum tomatoes, which are less watery than other tomato varieties. Canned whole plum tomatoes are also an option. The longer you keep the tomatoes roasting in the oven, the thicker and richer the sauce will become.

Green and White Pizza

Deanna traditionally makes this pizza with spinach and arugula, but the green topping possibilities are endless. Try out other combos, like zucchini with basil, asparagus with mint, or broccoli with basil. You can swap out the goat cheese for ricotta or the Parmesan for any aged cheese, such as Asiago or Romano.

SERVES

PREP TIME

COOK TIME

20

1 pound refrigerated fresh pizza dough

Nonstick cooking spray

2 tablespoons extra-virgin olive oil, divided

½ cup thinly sliced onion (about ¼ medium onion)

2 garlic cloves, minced (about 1 teaspoon)

3 cups baby spinach (about 3 ounces)

3 cups arugula (about 3 ounces)

¼ teaspoon freshly ground black pepper

1 tablespoon water

1 tablespoon freshly squeezed lemon juice (from ½ medium lemon)

All-purpose flour, for dusting

½ cup crumbled goat cheese (about 2 ounces)

½ cup shredded Parmesan cheese (about 2 ounces)

1. Preheat the oven to 500°F. Take the pizza dough out of the refrigerator. Coat a large, rimmed baking sheet with nonstick cooking spray.

2. In a large skillet over medium heat, heat 1 tablespoon of oil. Add the onion and cook for 4 minutes, stirring often. Add the garlic and cook for 1 minute, stirring often. Add the spinach, arugula, pepper, and water. Cook for about 2 minutes, stirring often, especially at the beginning, until all the greens are coated with oil and they start to cook down (they will shrink considerably). Remove the pan from the heat and mix in the lemon juice.

3. On a lightly floured surface, form the pizza dough into a 12-inch circle or a 10-by-12-inch rectangle, using a rolling pin or by stretching with your hands. Place the dough on the prepared baking sheet. Brush the dough with the remaining tablespoon of oil. Spread the cooked greens on top of the dough to within ½ inch of the edge. Crumble the goat cheese on top, then sprinkle with the Parmesan cheese.

CONTINUES NEXT PAGE

4. Bake for 10 to 12 minutes, or until the crust starts to brown around the edges. Remove from the oven, and slide the pizza onto a wooden cutting board. Cut into eight pieces with a pizza cutter or a sharp knife and serve.

Prep tip: In the summer, grill your pizza! Brush your cold grill with olive oil or spray with nonstick cooking spray, then heat to 500°F, or high heat. Brush the rolled-out dough with olive oil, and place the oiled side down on the grill grate. Then brush the side facing up with oil, cover with the grill lid, and let it cook for 2 to 3 minutes. Uncover and flip your crust with metal tongs or a spatula. Quickly add the toppings, then cover with the grill lid and cook for another 3 to 4 minutes, until the cheese is melted and the crust starts to look golden brown.

Per Serving Calories: 437; Total Fat: 17g; Saturated Fat: 7g; Cholesterol: 25mg; Sodium: 538mg; Total Carbohydrates: 56g; Fiber: 2g; Protein: 16g

White Clam Pizza Pie

NUT-FREE, EGG-FREE

SERVES

4

PREP
TIME

10

COOK
TIME

20

If you like spaghetti with clams, you'll love this garlicky pizza version of the classic shellfish pasta dish (even Deanna's tricky-eater husband loves it!). You don't need to fuss with fresh clams in their shells, as canned clams work beautifully in this dish, and we use the clam juice from the can for extra flavor. This pizza can also be made on the grill—check out our prep tip for Green and White Pizza (page 84) to see how.

1 pound refrigerated
fresh pizza dough

Nonstick cooking spray

2 tablespoons extra-virgin
olive oil, divided

2 garlic cloves, minced
(about 1 teaspoon)

½ teaspoon crushed
red pepper

1 (10-ounce) can whole
baby clams, drained,
⅓ cup of juice reserved

¼ cup dry white wine

All-purpose flour,
for dusting

1 cup diced fresh or
shredded mozzarella
cheese (about 4 ounces)

1 tablespoon grated
Pecorino Romano or
Parmesan cheese

1 tablespoon chopped fresh
flat-leaf (Italian) parsley

1. Preheat the oven to 500°F. Take the pizza dough out of the refrigerator. Coat a large, rimmed baking sheet with nonstick cooking spray.

2. In a large skillet over medium heat, heat 1½ tablespoons of the oil. Add the garlic and crushed red pepper and cook for 1 minute, stirring frequently to prevent the garlic from burning. Add the reserved clam juice and wine. Bring to a boil over high heat. Reduce to medium heat so the sauce is just simmering and cook for 10 minutes, stirring occasionally. The sauce will cook down and thicken.

3. Stir in the clams and cook for 3 minutes, stirring occasionally.

4. While the sauce is cooking, on a lightly floured surface, form the pizza dough into a 12-inch circle or into a 10-by-12-inch rectangle with a rolling pin or by stretching with your hands. Place the dough on the prepared baking sheet. Brush the dough with the remaining ½ tablespoon of oil. Set aside until the clam sauce is ready.

CONTINUES NEXT PAGE

5. Spread the clam sauce over the prepared dough within ½ inch of the edge. Top with the mozzarella cheese, then sprinkle with the Pecorino Romano.

6. Bake for 10 minutes, or until the crust starts to brown around the edges. Remove the pizza from the oven and slide onto a wooden cutting board. Top with the parsley, cut into eight pieces with a pizza cutter or a sharp knife, and serve.

Prep tip: To make a pizza for just one, divide the dough into four balls. Freeze three of the balls, wrapping each separately in plastic wrap and then adding them all to one large plastic zip-top freezer bag. Roll out the remaining dough ball and top your personal pizza, using one-fourth of the amounts of the toppings in the ingredients list.

Per Serving Calories: 541; Total Fat: 21g; Saturated Fat: 8g; Cholesterol: 62mg; Sodium: 583g; Total Carbohydrates: 56g; Fiber: 1g; Protein: 32g

Mediterranean Veggie Pizza with Pourable Thin Crust

NUT-FREE, VEGETARIAN, ONE POT

SERVES

4

PREP
TIME

15

COOK
TIME

15

In Serena's house, this easy-to-make pizza is a family favorite. It's just as good cold in lunch boxes (if you have any leftovers!). You can easily switch up the toppings; for example, thin zucchini slices could be baked into the crust instead of peppers. The eggs, whole-wheat flour, and cheese make this dish higher in protein—even without any meat.

Nonstick cooking spray

3 tablespoons cornmeal

1 cup white whole-wheat flour or regular whole-wheat flour

½ cup all-purpose flour

1 tablespoon dried oregano, crushed between your fingers

¼ teaspoon kosher or sea salt

1 cup plus 2 tablespoons 2% milk

2 large eggs, beaten

1 large bell pepper, sliced into ⅛-inch-thick rounds

1 (2.25-ounce) can sliced olives, any type of green or black, drained (about ½ cup)

3 whole canned artichoke hearts, drained and quartered

⅓ cup thinly sliced red onion (about ⅙ onion)

½ cup feta cheese (about 2 ounces), crumbled

Extra-virgin olive oil, for topping (optional)

CONTINUES NEXT PAGE

1. Place one oven rack about 4 inches below the broiler element. Preheat the oven to 400°F. Spray a large, rimmed baking sheet with nonstick cooking spray. Sprinkle it with the cornmeal and set aside.

2. In a large bowl, whisk together the flours, oregano, and salt. In a small bowl, whisk together the milk and eggs; mix into the flour mixture until well combined.

3. Pour the mixture onto the prepared baking sheet. Using a rubber scraper, carefully spread the batter evenly to the corners of the pan. Arrange the bell pepper slices evenly over the batter.

4. Bake on any oven rack for 10 to 12 minutes, or until the crust is dry on top. Remove the pizza crust from the oven.

5. Turn the oven broiler to high.

6. Top the pizza crust with the olives, artichoke hearts, and onion. Top with the feta cheese.

7. Place the pizza on the upper oven rack under the broiler. Broil until the cheese is melted and golden, rotating the pan halfway through and watching carefully to prevent burning. Top with a drizzle of olive oil.

Ingredient tip: We recommend using block feta cheese, not crumbled feta; block tastes much better and is not as dry and salty. Wash the block to remove even more salt before crumbling.

Per Serving Calories: 319; Total Fat: 10g; Saturated Fat: 5g; Cholesterol: 115mg; Sodium: 412mg; Total Carbohydrates: 47g; Fiber: 7g; Protein: 13g

Triple-Green Pasta

NUT-FREE, EGG-FREE, VEGETARIAN

SERVES

4

PREP
TIME

5

COOK
TIME

15

We use this recipe all year round to get a steaming pot of pasta with seasonal veggies on the table quickly. In summer, substitute chopped zucchini for the spinach, and in winter, try chopped kale or shredded cabbage. The trick is to undercook the pasta by about a minute so when it's added to the pan sauce, it soaks up all the flavors of the garlic and spices.

8 ounces uncooked penne

1 tablespoon
extra-virgin olive oil

2 garlic cloves, minced
(1 teaspoon)

¼ teaspoon crushed
red pepper

2 cups chopped fresh
flat-leaf (Italian) parsley,
including stems

5 cups loosely packed baby
spinach (about 5 ounces)

¼ teaspoon
ground nutmeg

¼ teaspoon freshly
ground black pepper

¼ teaspoon kosher
or sea salt

⅓ cup Castelvetrano olives
(or other green olives),
pitted and sliced (about 12)

⅓ cup grated Pecorino
Romano or Parmesan
cheese (about 1 ounce)

1. In a large stockpot, cook the pasta according to the package directions, but boil 1 minute less than instructed. Drain the pasta, and save ¼ cup of the cooking water.

2. While the pasta is cooking, in a large skillet over medium heat, heat the oil. Add the garlic and crushed red pepper, and cook for 30 seconds, stirring constantly. Add the parsley and cook for 1 minute, stirring constantly. Add the spinach, nutmeg, pepper, and salt, and cook for 3 minutes, stirring occasionally, until the spinach is wilted.

3. Add the pasta and the reserved ¼ cup pasta water to the skillet. Stir in the olives, and cook for about 2 minutes, until most of the pasta water has been absorbed. Remove from the heat, stir in the cheese, and serve.

Ingredient tip: Besides the multitude of pasta shapes on the market, there's also a huge variety when it comes to both wheat-based and wheat-free pastas. Whole-wheat, whole-grain, chickpea, lentil, quinoa, or a combination of grains and beans are all options. Our recommendation is to use the type of pasta you enjoy and pair it with vegetables, fish and seafood, and lean proteins, but also experiment with a new variety from time to time.

Per Serving Calories: 271; Total Fat: 8g; Saturated Fat: 2g; Cholesterol: 5mg; Sodium: 345mg; Total Carbohydrates: 43g; Fiber: 10g; Protein: 15g

No-Drain Pasta alla Norma

SERVES

6

PREP TIME

5

COOK TIME

25

You'll love Serena's no-drain shortcut to cooking pasta more quickly than the traditional method of waiting around for the water to boil. By using less water, the pasta cooking liquid turns into a thick sauce. Here, all the beloved Sicilian ingredients found in classic Pasta alla Norma—eggplant, tomatoes, basil, and cheese—simmer together in one pot right along with the pasta.

1 medium globe eggplant (about 1 pound), cut into ¾-inch cubes

1 tablespoon extra-virgin olive oil

1 cup chopped onion (about ½ medium onion)

8 ounces uncooked thin spaghetti

1 (15-ounce) container part-skim ricotta cheese

3 Roma tomatoes, chopped (about 2 cups)

2 garlic cloves, minced (about 1 teaspoon)

¼ teaspoon kosher or sea salt

½ cup loosely packed fresh basil leaves

Grated Parmesan cheese, for serving (optional)

1. Lay three paper towels on a large plate, and pile the cubed eggplant on top. (Don't cover the eggplant.) Microwave the eggplant on high for 5 minutes to dry and partially cook it.

2. In a large stockpot over medium-high heat, heat the oil. Add the eggplant and the onion and cook for 5 minutes, stirring occasionally.

3. Add the spaghetti, ricotta, tomatoes, garlic, and salt. Cover with water by a ½ inch (about 4 cups of water). Cook uncovered for 12 to 15 minutes, or until the pasta is just al dente (tender with a bite), stirring occasionally to prevent the pasta from sticking together or sticking to the bottom of the pot.

4. Remove the pot from the heat and let the pasta stand for 3 more minutes to absorb more liquid while you tear the basil into pieces. Sprinkle the basil over the pasta and gently stir. Serve with Parmesan cheese, if desired.

Prep tip: We use the microwave in this recipe to partially cook and moisten the eggplant, making it less spongy and less likely to sop up oil. We use a similar moistening trick in the Israeli Eggplant, Chickpea, and Mint Sauté (see page 58) by broiling the eggplant to make it silky smooth.

Per Serving Calories: 389; Total Fat: 9g; Saturated Fat: 4g; Cholesterol: 22mg; Sodium: 177mg; Total Carbohydrates: 62g; Fiber: 4g; Protein: 19g

Zucchini with Bow Ties

NUT-FREE, EGG-FREE, VEGETARIAN

Deanna's sister lived in Italy for four years. She picked up many cooking tips and authentic recipes like this one, which is a great way to use up extra zucchini during its peak season. Small pieces of zucchini are cooked down to a soft and silky pasta sauce and then mixed with a little milk and a generous amount of cheese.

3 tablespoons extra-virgin olive oil

2 garlic cloves, minced (about 1 teaspoon)

3 large or 4 medium zucchini, diced (about 4 cups)

½ teaspoon freshly ground black pepper

¼ teaspoon kosher or sea salt

½ cup 2% milk

¼ teaspoon ground nutmeg

8 ounces uncooked farfalle (bow ties) or other small pasta shape

½ cup grated Parmesan or Romano cheese (about 2 ounces)

1 tablespoon freshly squeezed lemon juice (from ½ medium lemon)

Per Serving Calories: 410; Total Fat: 17g; Saturated Fat: 4g; Cholesterol: 13mg; Sodium: 382mg; Total Carbohydrates: 45g; Fiber: 4g; Protein: 15g

1. In a large skillet over medium heat, heat the oil. Add the garlic and cook for 1 minute, stirring frequently. Add the zucchini, pepper, and salt. Stir well, cover, and cook for 15 minutes, stirring once or twice.

2. In a small, microwave-safe bowl, warm the milk in the microwave on high for 30 seconds. Stir the milk and nutmeg into the skillet and cook uncovered for another 5 minutes, stirring occasionally.

3. While the zucchini is cooking, in a large stockpot, cook the pasta according to the package directions.

4. Drain the pasta in a colander, saving about 2 tablespoons of pasta water. Add the pasta and pasta water to the skillet. Mix everything together and remove from the heat. Stir in the cheese and lemon juice and serve.

Prep tip: Did you know that a secret ingredient for bringing together a pasta sauce is pasta water? Save about ¼ to ½ cup of the starchy water before draining your cooked pasta. Add it to your sauce a few tablespoons at a time to thicken it up. Also, toss the pasta into the sauce right after draining to allow it to soak up more of the flavors of the sauce.

Roasted Asparagus Caprese Pasta

SERVES

6

PREP TIME

10

COOK TIME

15

This is Deanna's number one dish during asparagus season, as it's a great meal to whip up for a busy weeknight or for guests. The caprese part of this recipe refers to the combination of fresh mozzarella, tomatoes, and basil—a combo that supposedly originated on the Isle of Capri. When you can't get fresh asparagus, you can swap in just about any other veggie, such as broccoli, green beans, or zucchini.

8 ounces uncooked small pasta, like orecchiette (little ears) or farfalle (bow ties)

1½ pounds fresh asparagus, ends trimmed and stalks chopped into 1-inch pieces (about 3 cups)

1 pint grape tomatoes, halved (about 1½ cups)

2 tablespoons extra-virgin olive oil

¼ teaspoon freshly ground black pepper

¼ teaspoon kosher or sea salt

2 cups fresh mozzarella, drained and cut into bite-size pieces (about 8 ounces)

⅓ cup torn fresh basil leaves

2 tablespoons balsamic vinegar

1. Preheat the oven to 400°F.

2. In a large stockpot, cook the pasta according to the package directions. Drain, reserving about ¼ cup of the pasta water.

3. While the pasta is cooking, in a large bowl, toss the asparagus, tomatoes, oil, pepper, and salt together. Spread the mixture onto a large, rimmed baking sheet and bake for 15 minutes, stirring twice as it cooks.

4. Remove the vegetables from the oven, and add the cooked pasta to the baking sheet. Mix with a few tablespoons of pasta water to help the sauce become smoother and the saucy vegetables stick to the pasta.

5. Gently mix in the mozzarella and basil. Drizzle with the balsamic vinegar. Serve from the baking sheet or pour the pasta into a large bowl.

6. If you want to make this dish ahead of time or to serve it cold, follow the recipe up to step 4, then refrigerate the pasta and vegetables. When you are ready to serve, follow step 5 either with the cold pasta or with warm pasta that's been gently reheated in a pot on the stove.

Ingredient tip: If you have thicker and tougher asparagus stalks, use a knife to cut off about 1 inch of the tough stems. Or you can bend the stalks near the ends until they naturally snap in two; however, this method tends to waste more of the stalks. Either way, freeze those asparagus ends, along with other vegetable scraps like onion skins, kale stems, and carrot peels, to make homemade vegetable stock.

Per Serving Calories: 307; Total Fat: 14g; Saturated Fat: 6g; Cholesterol: 29mg; Sodium: 318mg; Total Carbohydrates: 33g; Fiber: 9g; Protein: 18g

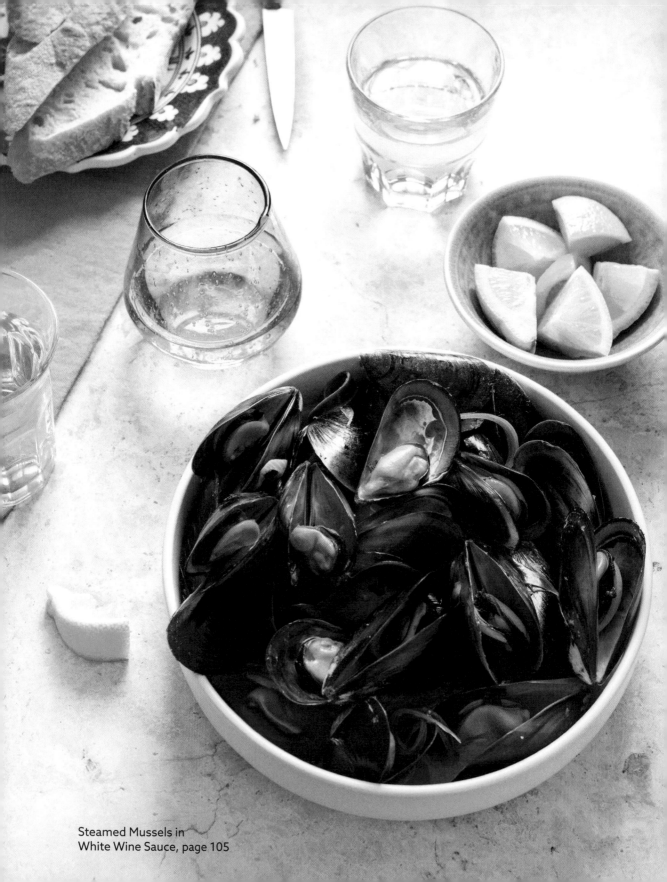

Steamed Mussels in
White Wine Sauce, page 105

EIGHT

Fish and Seafood

SINCE fish is a protein staple of the Mediterranean Diet, and because eating more of it brings so many health benefits (see chapter 1 to learn more about that), we made this the longest chapter in the book. Here you'll find 12 sensational recipes to get you hooked on seafood. From Crispy Polenta Fish Sticks (page 100) to Spicy Shrimp Puttanesca (page 109), we hope these dishes inspire and tempt you to eat the recommended two-plus fish servings per week.

Speedy Tilapia with Red Onion and Avocado

SERVES

PREP TIME

COOK TIME

5

DAIRY-FREE, NUT-FREE, GLUTEN-FREE, EGG-FREE,
5 INGREDIENTS, HALF THE TIME, ONE POT

We're pretty sure this recipe will change the way you think about preparing fish: perfectly cooked fillets in only 3 minutes . . . in the microwave! It works for almost any type of fish, and thanks to our folding trick, even uneven fillets (thicker at one end and thinner on the other) can be cooked this way. The result is super-tender, delicate fish fillets stuffed with citrusy onions and topped with creamy avocado.

1 tablespoon
extra-virgin olive oil

1 tablespoon freshly
squeezed orange juice

¼ teaspoon kosher
or sea salt

4 (4-ounce) tilapia fillets,
more oblong than square,
skin-on or skinned

¼ cup chopped red
onion (about ⅛ onion)

1 avocado, pitted,
skinned, and sliced

Per Serving Calories: 200;
Total Fat: 11g; Saturated Fat:
2g; Cholesterol: 55mg; Sodium:
161mg; Total Carbohydrates: 4g;
Fiber: 3g; Protein: 22g

1. In a 9-inch glass pie dish, use a fork to mix together the oil, orange juice, and salt. Working with one fillet at a time, place each in the pie dish and turn to coat on all sides. Arrange the fillets in a wagon-wheel formation, so that one end of each fillet is in the center of the dish and the other end is temporarily draped over the edge of the dish. Top each fillet with 1 tablespoon of onion, then fold the end of the fillet that's hanging over the edge in half over the onion. When finished, you should have 4 folded-over fillets with the fold against the outer edge of the dish and the ends all in the center.

2. Cover the dish with plastic wrap, leaving a small part open at the edge to vent the steam. Microwave on high for about 3 minutes. The fish is done when it just begins to separate into flakes (chunks) when pressed gently with a fork.

3. Top the fillets with the avocado and serve.

Prep tip: Because most fish skin is relatively thin, it cooks at about the same rate as fish flesh, which is why you can use this microwave method for both skin-on and skinless fish.

Grilled Fish on Lemons

DAIRY-FREE, NUT-FREE, GLUTEN-FREE, EGG-FREE, 5 INGREDIENTS, ONE POT

SERVES

4

PREP TIME

10

COOK TIME

10

It was 15 years into Serena's marriage before she attempted grilling—because her husband is really good at grilling, and why mess with a good thing? But this was the recipe hack that got Serena to take over the grilling tongs. Grilling fish on lemon slices infuses bright and smoky flavors fast and makes grill cleanup a snap.

4 (4-ounce) fish fillets, such as tilapia, salmon, catfish, cod, or your favorite fish

Nonstick cooking spray

3 to 4 medium lemons

1 tablespoon extra-virgin olive oil

¼ teaspoon freshly ground black pepper

¼ teaspoon kosher or sea salt

1. Using paper towels, pat the fillets dry and let stand at room temperature for 10 minutes. Meanwhile, coat the cold cooking grate of the grill with nonstick cooking spray, and preheat the grill to 400°F, or medium-high heat. Or preheat a grill pan over medium-high heat on the stove top.

2. Cut one lemon in half and set half aside. Slice the remaining half of that lemon and the remaining lemons into ¼-inch-thick slices. (You should have about 12 to 16 lemon slices.) Into a small bowl, squeeze 1 tablespoon of juice out of the reserved lemon half.

3. Add the oil to the bowl with the lemon juice, and mix well. Brush both sides of the fish with the oil mixture, and sprinkle evenly with pepper and salt.

CONTINUES NEXT PAGE

4. Carefully place the lemon slices on the grill (or the grill pan), arranging 3 to 4 slices together in the shape of a fish fillet, and repeat with the remaining slices. Place the fish fillets directly on top of the lemon slices, and grill with the lid closed. (If you're grilling on the stove top, cover with a large pot lid or aluminum foil.) Turn the fish halfway through the cooking time only if the fillets are more than half an inch thick. (See tip for cooking time.) The fish is done and ready to serve when it just begins to separate into flakes (chunks) when pressed gently with a fork.

Ingredient tip: We use the 10-minute-per-inch rule for grilling, baking, broiling, or panfrying any type of fish, since fish fillet sizes vary so much. Measure the thickest part of your fish fillets to determine the cooking time, and check the fish a minute or two before the suggested cooking time is up to prevent dried-out or overcooked fish. The fish is done when it just begins to separate into flakes (chunks) when pressed gently with a fork. The safe internal temperature for fish and seafood is 145°F.

Per Serving Calories: 147; Total Fat: 5g; Saturated Fat: 1g; Cholesterol: 55mg; Sodium: 158mg; Total Carbohydrates: 4g; Fiber: 1g; Protein: 22g

Weeknight Sheet Pan Fish Dinner

DAIRY-FREE, NUT-FREE, GLUTEN-FREE, EGG-FREE, 5 INGREDIENTS

This flavorful dish can be made with any fish fillet that is half an inch thick. And even though it's quick enough for a weeknight, it's such a colorful and delicious dish that Serena likes to serve it to guests as well. Fresh green beans are available most of the year, but when summer comes, be sure to make this with locally grown beans and tomatoes.

SERVES

4

PREP
TIME

10

COOK
TIME

10

Nonstick cooking spray

2 tablespoons extra-virgin olive oil

1 tablespoon balsamic vinegar

4 (4-ounce) fish fillets, such as cod or tilapia (½ inch thick)

2½ cups green beans (about 12 ounces)

1 pint cherry or grape tomatoes (about 2 cups)

Per Serving Calories: 193; Total Fat: 8g; Saturated Fat: 2g; Cholesterol: 55mg; Sodium: 49mg; Total Carbohydrates: 8g; Fiber: 3g; Protein: 23g

1. Preheat the oven to 400°F. Coat two large, rimmed baking sheets with nonstick cooking spray.

2. In a small bowl, whisk together the oil and vinegar. Set aside.

3. Place two pieces of fish on each baking sheet.

4. In a large bowl, combine the beans and tomatoes. Pour in the oil and vinegar, and toss gently to coat. Pour half of the green bean mixture over the fish on one baking sheet, and the remaining half over the fish on the other. Turn the fish over, and rub it in the oil mixture to coat. Spread the vegetables evenly on the baking sheets so hot air can circulate around them.

5. Bake for 5 to 8 minutes, until the fish is just opaque and not translucent. The fish is done and ready to serve when it just begins to separate into flakes (chunks) when pressed gently with a fork.

Prep tip: To ensure that the fish cooks evenly, fold under any thin sections of the fillets so the entire fillet is half an inch thick.

Crispy Polenta Fish Sticks

NUT-FREE

SERVES

4

PREP TIME

15

COOK TIME

10

Polenta is an Italian favorite that is essentially cooked cornmeal mush; it's often used as the base starch over which to spoon savory sauces and stews. Here we used regular cornmeal to add big-time crunch and sweet corn flavor to these baked fish sticks. One of Serena's daughters doesn't usually like fish, but she will ask for seconds of these dippable, fun fish sticks. Serve them with the creamy yogurt tzatziki sauce from our Chickpea Patties in Pitas recipe (page 75, step 3).

2 large eggs, lightly beaten

1 tablespoon 2% milk

1 pound skinned fish fillets (cod, tilapia, or other white fish) about ½ inch thick, sliced into 20 (1-inch-wide) strips

½ cup yellow cornmeal

½ cup whole-wheat panko bread crumbs or whole-wheat bread crumbs

¼ teaspoon smoked paprika

¼ teaspoon kosher or sea salt

¼ teaspoon freshly ground black pepper

Nonstick cooking spray

Per Serving Calories: 256; Total Fat: 6g; Saturated Fat: 1g; Cholesterol: 148mg; Sodium: 321mg; Total Carbohydrates: 22g; Fiber: 2g; Protein: 29g

1. Place a large, rimmed baking sheet in the oven. Preheat the oven to 400°F with the pan inside.

2. In a large bowl, mix the eggs and milk. Using a fork, add the fish strips to the egg mixture and stir gently to coat.

3. Put the cornmeal, bread crumbs, smoked paprika, salt, and pepper in a quart-size zip-top plastic bag. Using a fork or tongs, transfer the fish to the bag, letting the excess egg wash drip off into the bowl before transferring. Seal the bag and shake gently to completely coat each fish stick.

4. With oven mitts, carefully remove the hot baking sheet from the oven and spray it with nonstick cooking spray. Using a fork or tongs, remove the fish sticks from the bag and arrange them on the hot baking sheet, with space between them so the hot air can circulate and crisp them up.

5. Bake for 5 to 8 minutes, until gentle pressure with a fork causes the fish to flake, and serve.

Prep tip: The hands-free technique we use above to batter the fish is no-mess and works well for smaller fish sticks or chicken nuggets. Using a fork and coating the fish inside a bag keeps your fingers from getting messy and covered with batter.

Salmon Skillet Supper

DAIRY-FREE, NUT-FREE, GLUTEN-FREE, EGG-FREE, ONE POT

This fish dish has it all: tons of flavor; it cooks in one pot; it's nutrient-packed with omega-3s, vitamins A, C, D, and E, fiber, and potassium; and you can serve it many different ways. Enjoy it as is, or spoon it over rice, pasta, or your favorite whole grain. It's still tasty the next day, when you can stuff the fish and saucy vegetables into a pita pocket or heat them up for a protein-packed start to the morning. Who says you can't have salmon for breakfast?

1 tablespoon
extra-virgin olive oil

2 garlic cloves, minced
(about 1 teaspoon)

1 teaspoon smoked paprika

1 pint grape or cherry
tomatoes, quartered
(about 1½ cups)

1 (12-ounce) jar roasted
red peppers, drained
and chopped

1 tablespoon water

¼ teaspoon freshly
ground black pepper

¼ teaspoon kosher
or sea salt

1 pound salmon fillets, skin
removed, cut into 8 pieces

1 tablespoon freshly
squeezed lemon juice
(from ½ medium lemon)

1. In a large skillet over medium heat, heat the oil. Add the garlic and smoked paprika and cook for 1 minute, stirring often. Add the tomatoes, roasted peppers, water, black pepper, and salt. Turn up the heat to medium-high, bring to a simmer, and cook for 3 minutes, stirring occasionally and smashing the tomatoes with a wooden spoon toward the end of the cooking time.

2. Add the salmon to the skillet, and spoon some of the sauce over the top. Cover and cook for 10 to 12 minutes, or until the salmon is cooked through (145°F using a meat thermometer) and just starts to flake.

3. Remove the skillet from the heat, and drizzle lemon juice over the top of the fish. Stir the sauce, then break up the salmon into chunks with a fork. You can serve it straight from the skillet.

Per Serving Calories: 289; Total Fat: 13g; Saturated Fat: 2g; Cholesterol: 68mg; Sodium: 393mg; Total Carbohydrates: 10g; Fiber: 2g; Protein: 31g

Prep tip: There's a lot of confusion about wild vs. farm-raised fish, but the bottom line is that both fishing practices can be sustainable. These days, both wild and farmed fish are often harvested responsibly, meaning they have a minimal impact on the environment. To keep up to date on the best sustainable seafood choices on the market today, visit FishWatch.gov.

Tuscan Tuna and Zucchini Burgers

SERVES

4

PREP
TIME

10

COOK
TIME

10

Serena had a lot of tuna burger fails before she got this recipe just right. You'll love these burgers with crispy, crunchy crusts and thick, juicy centers. Not only do the bright specks of sweet red pepper look pretty, but they also pair well with the lemon zest and savory oregano. Most importantly, this recipe is a winner because these burgers won't fall apart when you flip them.

3 slices whole-wheat sandwich bread, toasted

2 (5-ounce) cans tuna in olive oil, drained

1 cup shredded zucchini (about ¾ small zucchini)

1 large egg, lightly beaten

¼ cup diced red bell pepper (about ¼ pepper)

1 tablespoon dried oregano

1 teaspoon lemon zest

¼ teaspoon freshly ground black pepper

¼ teaspoon kosher or sea salt

1 tablespoon extra-virgin olive oil

Salad greens or 4 whole-wheat rolls, for serving (optional)

Per Serving Calories: 191; Total Fat: 10g; Saturated Fat: 2g; Cholesterol: 72mg; Sodium: 472mg; Total Carbohydrates: 11g; Fiber: 2g; Protein: 15g

1. Crumble the toast into bread crumbs using your fingers (or use a knife to cut into ¼-inch cubes) until you have 1 cup of loosely packed crumbs. Pour the crumbs into a large bowl. Add the tuna, zucchini, egg, bell pepper, oregano, lemon zest, black pepper, and salt. Mix well with a fork. With your hands, form the mixture into four (½-cup-size) patties. Place on a plate, and press each patty flat to about ¾-inch thick.

2. In a large skillet over medium-high heat, heat the oil until it's very hot, about 2 minutes. Add the patties to the hot oil, then turn the heat down to medium. Cook the patties for 5 minutes, flip with a spatula, and cook for an additional 5 minutes. Enjoy as is or serve on salad greens or whole-wheat rolls.

Ingredient tip: Think of black pepper as a spice, not just a partner to salt. Black pepper can perk up a dish with a bit of heat, but without overwhelming other flavors. For the best flavor, buy whole peppercorns and grind them in a pepper mill or coffee grinder. Or buy the plastic mills that already contain whole peppercorns (in the spice aisle).

Sicilian Kale and Tuna Bowl

SERVES

PREP TIME

COOK TIME

15

Sadly, canned tuna is often relegated to sandwiches and the occasional casserole. Hopefully, this robust recipe with greens will get you thinking about using canned tuna in more varied ways. It's tangy, sweet, briny, spicy—and all cooked in one pot.

1 pound kale, chopped, center ribs removed (about 12 cups)

3 tablespoons extra-virgin olive oil

1 cup chopped onion (about ½ medium onion)

3 garlic cloves, minced (about 1½ teaspoons)

1 (2.25-ounce) can sliced olives, drained (about ½ cup)

¼ cup capers

¼ teaspoon crushed red pepper

2 teaspoons sugar

2 (6-ounce) cans tuna in olive oil, undrained

1 (15-ounce) can cannellini beans or great northern beans, drained and rinsed

¼ teaspoon freshly ground black pepper

¼ teaspoon kosher or sea salt

1. Fill a large stockpot three-quarters full of water, and bring to a boil. Add the kale and cook for 2 minutes. (This is to make the kale less bitter.) Drain the kale in a colander and set aside.

2. Set the empty pot back on the stove over medium heat, and pour in the oil. Add the onion and cook for 4 minutes, stirring often. Add the garlic and cook for 1 minute, stirring often. Add the olives, capers, and crushed red pepper, and cook for 1 minute, stirring often. Add the partially cooked kale and sugar, stirring until the kale is completely coated with oil. Cover the pot and cook for 8 minutes.

3. Remove the kale from the heat, mix in the tuna, beans, pepper, and salt, and serve.

Prep tip: Thick, dark, leafy veggies like kale, Swiss chard, and collard greens can be intimidating to prepare. The key is to remove the stems or ribs. Layer three to four leaves on top of each other and fold in half. Run your knife right along the side of the thick stem to remove it completely. Chop the remaining leaves for your recipe and compost the stems (or save in the freezer to make vegetable stock).

Per Serving Calories: 265; Total Fat: 12g; Saturated Fat: 2g; Cholesterol: 21mg; Sodium: 710mg; Total Carbohydrates: 26g; Fiber: 7g; Protein: 16g

Mediterranean Cod Stew

SERVES

6

PREP TIME

10

COOK TIME

20

This robust seafood stew, featuring buttery cod, sweet tomatoes, meaty mushrooms, and fruity olives, is a less labor-intensive variation of traditional fish stews like cioppino and bouillabaisse. We like to pair it with a fresh salad, like our Easy Italian Orange and Celery Salad (page 41), and a loaf of crusty bread.

2 tablespoons extra-virgin olive oil

2 cups chopped onion (about 1 medium onion)

2 garlic cloves, minced (about 1 teaspoon)

¾ teaspoon smoked paprika

1 (14.5-ounce) can diced tomatoes, undrained

1 (12-ounce) jar roasted red peppers, drained and chopped

1 cup sliced olives, green or black

⅓ cup dry red wine

¼ teaspoon freshly ground black pepper

¼ teaspoon kosher or sea salt

1½ pounds cod fillets, cut into 1-inch pieces

3 cups sliced mushrooms (about 8 ounces)

1. In a large stockpot over medium heat, heat the oil. Add the onion and cook for 4 minutes, stirring occasionally. Add the garlic and smoked paprika and cook for 1 minute, stirring often.

2. Mix in the tomatoes with their juices, roasted peppers, olives, wine, pepper, and salt, and turn the heat up to medium-high. Bring to a boil. Add the cod and mushrooms, and reduce the heat to medium.

3. Cover and cook for about 10 minutes, stirring a few times, until the cod is cooked through and flakes easily, and serve.

Ingredient tip: If your recipe calls for wine and you don't have any on hand, here are some substitutions. For sweet white or red wine, use equal amounts of apple juice or grape juice. For dry white or red wine, swap in equal amounts of chicken or vegetable broth. Also, try 1 tablespoon of lemon juice or white wine vinegar mixed with ½ cup of water (for white wine) or 1 tablespoon of red wine vinegar mixed with ½ cup of water (for red wine).

Per Serving Calories: 220; Total Fat: 8g; Saturated Fat: 1g; Cholesterol: 55mg; Sodium: 474mg; Total Carbohydrates: 12g; Fiber: 3g; Protein: 28g

Steamed Mussels in White Wine Sauce

DAIRY-FREE, NUT-FREE, GLUTEN-FREE, EGG-FREE, ONE POT, HALF THE TIME

SERVES

4

PREP TIME

5

COOK TIME

10

Serena used to think mussels were too "fancy" to prepare at home. Then she got the courage to order some from the friendly fishmonger at her local supermarket. Mussels are so easy to cook. Just a few minutes in the pot, and you've got an amazingly tasty, inexpensive, and sustainable seafood dinner. Serve them with crusty bread to sop up the garlicky, lemony broth.

2 pounds small mussels

1 tablespoon extra-virgin olive oil

1 cup thinly sliced red onion (about ½ medium onion)

3 garlic cloves, sliced (about 1½ teaspoons)

1 cup dry white wine

2 (¼-inch-thick) lemon slices

¼ teaspoon freshly ground black pepper

¼ teaspoon kosher or sea salt

Fresh lemon wedges, for serving (optional)

1. In a large colander in the sink, run cold water over the mussels (but don't let the mussels sit in standing water). All the shells should be closed tight; discard any shells that are a little bit open or any shells that are cracked. Leave the mussels in the colander until you're ready to use them.

2. In a large skillet over medium-high heat, heat the oil. Add the onion and cook for 4 minutes, stirring occasionally. Add the garlic and cook for 1 minute, stirring constantly. Add the wine, lemon slices, pepper, and salt, and bring to a simmer. Cook for 2 minutes.

3. Add the mussels and cover. Cook for 3 minutes, or until the mussels open their shells. Gently shake the pan two or three times while they are cooking.

CONTINUES NEXT PAGE

4. All the shells should now be wide open. Using a slotted spoon, discard any mussels that are still closed. Spoon the opened mussels into a shallow serving bowl, and pour the broth over the top. Serve with additional fresh lemon slices, if desired.

Prep tip: About the only way you can mess up mussels is by drowning them. Remember, they're still alive, so they need to breathe. Ask your fishmonger to put a little ice in the box with your mussels. When you get home, dump out the melted ice, put the mussels in the refrigerator, and cook them within 24 hours.

Per Serving Calories: 222; Total Fat: 7g; Saturated Fat: 1g; Cholesterol: 42mg; Sodium: 547mg; Total Carbohydrates: 11g; Fiber: 1g; Protein: 18g

Orange and Garlic Shrimp

DAIRY-FREE, NUT-FREE, GLUTEN-FREE, EGG-FREE, ONE POT

Sautéed in a pan in the winter or thrown on the grill in the summer, this superb shrimp dish is a winner in any season. While testing out the recipe for this cookbook, Deanna decided to add in orange segments, and now this is her favorite way to serve it.

1 large orange

3 tablespoons extra-virgin olive oil, divided

1 tablespoon chopped fresh rosemary (about 3 sprigs) or 1 teaspoon dried rosemary

1 tablespoon chopped fresh thyme (about 6 sprigs) or 1 teaspoon dried thyme

3 garlic cloves, minced (about 1½ teaspoons)

¼ teaspoon freshly ground black pepper

¼ teaspoon kosher or sea salt

1½ pounds fresh raw shrimp, (or frozen and thawed raw shrimp) shells and tails removed

Per Serving Calories: 190; Total Fat: 8g; Saturated Fat: 1g; Cholesterol: 221mg; Sodium: 215mg; Total Carbohydrates: 4g; Fiber: 1g; Protein: 24g

1. Zest the entire orange using a Microplane or citrus grater.

2. In a large zip-top plastic bag, combine the orange zest and 2 tablespoons of oil with the rosemary, thyme, garlic, pepper, and salt. Add the shrimp, seal the bag, and gently massage the shrimp until all the ingredients are combined and the shrimp is completely covered with the seasonings. Set aside.

3. Heat a grill, grill pan, or a large skillet over medium heat. Brush on or swirl in the remaining 1 tablespoon of oil. Add half the shrimp, and cook for 4 to 6 minutes, or until the shrimp turn pink and white, flipping halfway through if on the grill or stirring every minute if in a pan. Transfer the shrimp to a large serving bowl. Repeat with the remaining shrimp, and add them to the bowl.

4. While the shrimp cook, peel the orange and cut the flesh into bite-size pieces. Add to the serving bowl, and toss with the cooked shrimp. Serve immediately or refrigerate and serve cold.

Ingredient tip: For different flavor combinations, try lemon zest instead of the orange zest and ¼ cup chopped fresh mint instead of rosemary and thyme, or lime zest instead of the orange zest and ¼ to ½ teaspoon crushed red pepper instead of the thyme.

Roasted Shrimp-Gnocchi Bake

SERVES
4

PREP TIME
10

COOK TIME
20

This dish is one of Deanna's go-to weeknight dinners to get more seafood into her family's meals, because she usually has shrimp and gnocchi in her freezer. Occasionally she swaps in other varieties of small pasta, like farfalle (bow ties), fusilli (twisters), or orecchiette (little ears) for the gnocchi.

1 cup chopped fresh tomato (about 1 large tomato)

2 tablespoons extra-virgin olive oil

2 garlic cloves, minced (about 1 teaspoon)

½ teaspoon freshly ground black pepper

¼ teaspoon crushed red pepper

1 (12-ounce) jar roasted red peppers, drained and coarsely chopped

1 pound fresh raw shrimp (or frozen and thawed shrimp), shells and tails removed

1 pound frozen gnocchi (not thawed)

½ cup cubed feta cheese (about 2 ounces)

⅓ cup fresh torn basil leaves

1. Preheat the oven to 425°F.

2. In a baking dish, mix the tomatoes, oil, garlic, black pepper, and crushed red pepper. Roast in the oven for 10 minutes.

3. Stir in the roasted peppers and shrimp. Roast for 10 more minutes, until the shrimp turn pink and white.

4. While the shrimp cooks, cook the gnocchi on the stove top according to the package directions. Drain in a colander and keep warm.

5. Remove the dish from the oven. Mix in the cooked gnocchi, feta, and basil, and serve.

Ingredient tip: You can substitute drained canned diced tomatoes for the chopped tomatoes. Look for low-sodium or no-salt-added canned tomatoes.

Per Serving Calories: 277; Total Fat: 7g; Saturated Fat: 2g; Cholesterol: 130mg; Sodium: 653mg; Total Carbohydrates: 35g; Fiber: 1g; Protein: 20g

Spicy Shrimp Puttanesca

DAIRY-FREE, NUT-FREE, GLUTEN-FREE, EGG-FREE, ONE POT

SERVES

4

PREP
TIME

5

COOK
TIME

15

If you like a kick to your seafood, this classic Italian spicy sauce is for you. Don't let the anchovies hold you back—these tiny fish actually melt into the sauce, giving it a meaty flavor without a fishy taste. For a pop of green and an extra veggie boost, stir in 2 cups of spinach or arugula during the last minute of cooking.

2 tablespoons
extra-virgin olive oil

3 anchovy fillets,
drained and chopped
(half a 2-ounce tin),
or 1½ teaspoons
anchovy paste

3 garlic cloves, minced
(about 1½ teaspoons)

½ teaspoon crushed
red pepper

1 (14.5-ounce) can
low-sodium or
no-salt-added diced
tomatoes, undrained

1 (2.25-ounce) can
sliced black olives,
drained (about ½ cup)

2 tablespoons capers

1 tablespoon chopped
fresh oregano or
1 teaspoon dried oregano

1 pound fresh raw
shrimp (or frozen and
thawed shrimp), shells
and tails removed

1. In a large skillet over medium heat, heat the oil. Mix in the anchovies, garlic, and crushed red pepper. Cook for 3 minutes, stirring frequently and mashing up the anchovies with a wooden spoon, until they have melted into the oil.

2. Stir in the tomatoes with their juices, olives, capers, and oregano. Turn up the heat to medium-high, and bring to a simmer.

3. When the sauce is lightly bubbling, stir in the shrimp. Reduce the heat to medium, and cook the shrimp for 6 to 8 minutes, or until they turn pink and white, stirring occasionally, and serve.

Ingredient tip: When buying anchovies to use as a recipe flavor enhancer, there are two convenient options: canned anchovies packed in oil in 2-ounce tins or anchovy paste, sold in 2-ounce tubes. Both items are high in sodium, but the good news is that using just a small amount gives a strong, meaty taste to recipes—and you won't need to add any salt to your dish.

Per Serving Calories: 214; Total Fat: 10g; Saturated Fat: 2g; Cholesterol: 178mg; Sodium: 553mg; Total Carbohydrates: 7g; Fiber: 2g; Protein: 26g

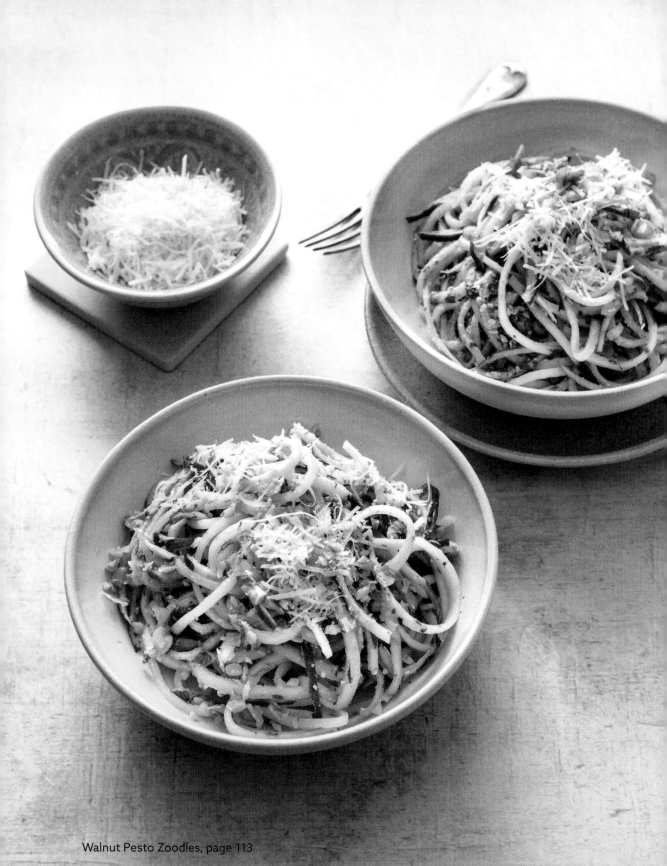

Walnut Pesto Zoodles, page 113

NINE

Vegetable Main Dishes

WE'VE packed this chapter with vibrant, veggie-forward dishes that even a carnivore will love. The key to making vegetarian and vegan meals ultra-appealing the Mediterranean way is to cook the veggies just right, and then enhance them with super-flavorful staples like buttery olive oil, aged cheeses, rich nuts, fresh herbs, and bold spices. From Gorgonzola Sweet Potato Burgers (page 118) to Polenta with Mushroom Bolognese (page 126), we promise you'll leave the table feeling satisfied and happy

Greek Stuffed Collard Greens

NUT-FREE, GLUTEN-FREE, EGG-FREE, VEGETARIAN, 5 INGREDIENTS

SERVES

4

PREP TIME

10

COOK TIME

20

Here's our riff on the traditional rice-stuffed grape leaves, using more manageable and easier-to-find collard greens and our Mediterranean Lentils and Rice recipe (page 60) as the savory stuffing.

1 (28-ounce) can low-sodium or no-salt-added crushed tomatoes

8 collard green leaves (about ⅓ pound), tough tips of stems cut off

1 recipe Mediterranean Lentils and Rice (page 60) or 2 (10-ounce) bags frozen grain medley (about 4 cups), cooked

2 tablespoons grated Parmesan cheese

Per Serving Calories: 205; Total Fat: 8g; Saturated Fat: 2g; Cholesterol: 3mg; Sodium: 524mg; Total Carbohydrates: 34g; Fiber: 8g; Protein: 6g

1. Preheat the oven to 400°F. Pour the tomatoes into a baking pan and set aside.

2. Fill a large stockpot about three-quarters of the way with water and bring to a boil. Add the collard greens and cook for 2 minutes. Drain in a colander. Put the greens on a clean towel or paper towels and blot dry.

3. To assemble the stuffed collards, lay one leaf flat on the counter vertically. Add about ½ cup of the lentils and rice mixture to the middle of the leaf, and spread it evenly along the middle of the leaf. Fold one long side of the leaf over the rice filling, then fold over the other long side so it is slightly overlapping. Take the bottom end, where the stem was, and gently but firmly roll up until you have a slightly square package. Carefully transfer the stuffed leaf to the baking pan, and place it seam-side down in the crushed tomatoes. Repeat with the remaining leaves.

4. Sprinkle the leaves with the grated cheese, and cover the pan with aluminum foil. Bake for 20 minutes, or until the collards are tender-firm, and serve. (If you prefer softer greens, bake for an additional 10 minutes.)

Ingredient tip: Instead of collard greens, you can use partially boiled cabbage leaves or raw romaine leaves. Or, if you're feeling adventurous, use jarred grape leaves, which you may find in the international aisle at your grocery store.

Walnut Pesto Zoodles

GLUTEN-FREE, EGG-FREE, VEGETARIAN, ONE POT

SERVES

4

PREP TIME

15

COOK TIME

10

Being a lifelong pasta eater, Deanna was slow to jump on the veggie "noodle" bandwagon. She didn't feel the need to give up her beloved spaghetti. She finally broke down and bought a spiralizer last summer to help prepare the glut of zucchini she was getting in her CSA share. Now she's a convert—not to completely substituting veggies for pasta, but rather to adding more spiralized vegetables into lots of dishes with this easy kitchen tool.

4 medium zucchini (makes about 8 cups of zoodles)

¼ cup extra-virgin olive oil, divided

2 garlic cloves, minced (about 1 teaspoon), divided

½ teaspoon crushed red pepper

¼ teaspoon freshly ground black pepper, divided

¼ teaspoon kosher or sea salt, divided

2 tablespoons grated Parmesan cheese, divided

1 cup packed fresh basil leaves

¾ cup walnut pieces, divided

1. Make the zucchini noodles (zoodles) using a spiralizer or your vegetable peeler to make ribbons (run the peeler down the zucchini to make long strips). In a large bowl, gently mix to combine the zoodles with 1 tablespoon of oil, 1 minced garlic clove, all the crushed red pepper, ⅛ teaspoon of black pepper, and ⅛ teaspoon of salt. Set aside.

2. In a large skillet over medium-high heat, heat ½ tablespoon of oil. Add half of the zoodles to the pan and cook for 5 minutes, stirring every minute or so. Pour the cooked zoodles into a large serving bowl, and repeat with another ½ tablespoon of oil and the remaining zoodles. Add those zoodles to the serving bowl when they are done cooking.

CONTINUES NEXT PAGE

3. While the zoodles are cooking, make the pesto. If you're using a food processor, add the remaining minced garlic clove, ⅛ teaspoon of black pepper, and ⅛ teaspoon of salt, 1 tablespoon of Parmesan, all the basil leaves, and ¼ cup of walnuts. Turn on the processor, and slowly drizzle the remaining 2 tablespoons of oil into the opening until the pesto is completely blended. If you're using a high-powered blender, add the 2 tablespoons of oil first and then the rest of the pesto ingredients. Pulse until the pesto is completely blended.

4. Add the pesto to the zoodles along with the remaining 1 tablespoon of Parmesan and the remaining ½ cup of walnuts. Mix together well and serve.

Ingredient tip: By using your food processor or high-powered blender, homemade pesto is just a few pulses away. Traditional pesto calls for basil leaves and pine nuts, but we've substituted many flavorful combinations of greens, like arugula, mint, cilantro, and parsley, along with different nuts like pecans, walnuts, pistachios, and almonds to make a variety of vibrant pestos. To make your pesto bright green, Serena recommends using leafy green carrot tops (yes, really!) for half the amount of greens called for in the pesto recipe. Freeze any extra pesto you may have in an ice cube tray, then pop the cubes into a plastic freezer bag for use in soups and stews.

Per Serving Calories: 301; Total Fat: 28g; Saturated Fat: 4g; Cholesterol: 3mg; Sodium: 170mg; Total Carbohydrates: 11g; Fiber: 4g; Protein: 7g

Cauliflower Steaks with Eggplant Relish

SERVES

4

PREP
TIME

5

COOK
TIME

25

NUT-FREE, GLUTEN-FREE, VEGAN, 5 INGREDIENTS

These thick slabs of golden roasted cauliflower are substantial enough to serve as a hearty vegan main. Serena's kids now specifically request these "yummy big cauliflowers," then slather them with ketchup. We like to slather them with Eggplant Relish Spread (page 33) and serve them with typical steak sides, like sautéed mushrooms, baked potatoes, and Caesar salad.

2 small heads cauliflower (about 3 pounds)

¼ teaspoon kosher or sea salt

¼ teaspoon smoked paprika

extra-virgin olive oil, divided

1 recipe Eggplant Relish Spread (page 33) or 1 container store-bought baba ghanoush

1. Place a large, rimmed baking sheet in the oven. Preheat the oven to 400°F with the pan inside.

2. Stand one head of cauliflower on a cutting board, stem-end down. With a long chef's knife, slice down through the very center of the head, including the stem. Starting at the cut edge, measure about 1 inch and cut one thick slice from each cauliflower half, including as much of the stem as possible, to make two cauliflower "steaks." Reserve the remaining cauliflower for another use. Repeat with the second cauliflower head.

3. Dry each steak well with a clean towel. Sprinkle the salt and smoked paprika evenly over both sides of each cauliflower steak.

CONTINUES NEXT PAGE

4. In a large skillet over medium-high heat, heat 2 tablespoons of oil. When the oil is very hot, add two cauliflower steaks to the pan and cook for about 3 minutes, until golden and crispy. Flip and cook for 2 more minutes. Transfer the steaks to a plate. Use a pair of tongs to hold a paper towel and wipe out the pan to remove most of the hot oil (which will contain a few burnt bits of cauliflower). Repeat the cooking process with the remaining 2 tablespoons of oil and the remaining two steaks.

5. Using oven mitts, carefully remove the baking sheet from the oven and place the cauliflower on the baking sheet. Roast in the oven for 12 to 15 minutes, until the cauliflower steaks are just fork tender; they will still be somewhat firm. Serve the steaks with the Eggplant Relish Spread, baba ghanoush, or the homemade ketchup from our Italian Baked Beans recipe (page 56).

Ingredient tip: Smoked paprika, a staple in Spanish cuisine, is one of our favorite go-to spices. Made from dried smoked peppers that have been ground into a powder, it adds a lovely, sweet, smoky flavor with a kick of heat. It's a terrific substitute for bacon, ham, or other smoked meats in vegetarian dishes.

Per Serving Calories: 282; Total Fat: 22g; Saturated Fat: 3g; Cholesterol: 7mg; Sodium: 380mg; Total Carbohydrates: 20g; Fiber: 9g; Protein: 8g

Mediterranean Lentil Sloppy Joes

NUT-FREE, VEGAN, ONE POT

This family-favorite meal is quick, simple, and less messy than the original Sloppy Joes, since much neater pita pockets replace hamburger buns. This recipe was one of our most tested and was heartily approved by both meat lovers and vegetarians.

SERVES

4

PREP TIME

5

COOK TIME

15

1 tablespoon extra-virgin olive oil

1 cup chopped onion (about ½ medium onion)

1 cup chopped bell pepper, any color (about 1 medium bell pepper)

2 garlic cloves, minced (about 1 teaspoon)

1 (15-ounce) can lentils, drained and rinsed

1 (14.5-ounce) can low-sodium or no-salt-added diced tomatoes, undrained

1 teaspoon ground cumin

1 teaspoon dried thyme

¼ teaspoon kosher or sea salt

4 whole-wheat pita breads, split open

1½ cups chopped seedless cucumber (1 medium cucumber)

1 cup chopped romaine lettuce

1. In a medium saucepan over medium-high heat, heat the oil. Add the onion and bell pepper and cook for 4 minutes, stirring frequently. Add the garlic and cook for 1 minute, stirring frequently. Add the lentils, tomatoes (with their liquid), cumin, thyme, and salt. Turn the heat to medium and cook, stirring occasionally, for 10 minutes, or until most of the liquid has evaporated.

2. Stuff the lentil mixture inside each pita. Lay the cucumbers and lettuce on top of the lentil mixture and serve.

Ingredient tip: Using dry brown lentils is also an option for this recipe. After cooking the garlic, add ¾ cup dried lentils and 2¼ cups water, cover, and cook on medium heat for 15 minutes. Add the rest of the ingredients in step 1, cover again, and cook on medium heat for another 15 minutes, or until most of the liquid has evaporated.

Per Serving Calories: 334; Total Fat: 5g; Saturated Fat: 1g; Cholesterol: 0mg; Sodium: 610mg; Total Carbohydrates: 58g; Fiber: 10g; Protein: 16g

Gorgonzola Sweet Potato Burgers

NUT-FREE, VEGETARIAN, ONE POT

These thick, juicy veggie burgers are stuffed with the appealing combination of sweet potatoes and tangy blue cheese. We like to serve them on a plate of green salad that's been dressed with lemon juice and olive oil, but they're also super yummy inside a toasted whole-wheat roll, with a thick slice of red onion.

1 large sweet potato
(about 8 ounces)

2 tablespoons extra-virgin
olive oil, divided

1 cup chopped onion
(about ½ medium onion)

1 cup old-fashioned
rolled oats

1 large egg

1 tablespoon
balsamic vinegar

1 tablespoon dried oregano

1 garlic clove

¼ teaspoon kosher
or sea salt

½ cup crumbled
Gorgonzola or blue
cheese (about 2 ounces)

Salad greens or
4 whole-wheat rolls,
for serving (optional)

1. Using a fork, pierce the sweet potato all over and microwave on high for 4 to 5 minutes, until tender in the center. Cool slightly, then slice in half.

2. While the sweet potato is cooking, in a large skillet over medium-high heat, heat 1 tablespoon of oil. Add the onion and cook for 5 minutes, stirring occasionally.

3. Using a spoon, carefully scoop the sweet potato flesh out of the skin and put the flesh in a food processor. Add the onion, oats, egg, vinegar, oregano, garlic, and salt. Process until smooth. Add the cheese and pulse four times to barely combine. With your hands, form the mixture into four (½-cup-size) burgers. Place the burgers on a plate, and press to flatten each to about ¾-inch thick.

4. Wipe out the skillet with a paper towel, then heat the remaining 1 tablespoon of oil over medium-high heat until very hot, about 2 minutes. Add the burgers to the hot oil, then turn the heat down to medium. Cook the burgers for 5 minutes, flip with a spatula, then cook an additional 5 minutes. Enjoy as is or serve on salad greens or whole-wheat rolls.

Prep tip: To make your burgers a uniform size, divide the burger mixture into roughly quarter sections, then pack a portion into a ½-cup measuring cup. Pop each burger out of the measuring cup, then flatten and pack it with your hands into a ¾-inch-thick patty.

Per Serving Calories: 223; Total Fat: 13g; Saturated Fat: 4g; Cholesterol: 60mg; Sodium: 330mg; Total Carbohydrates: 21g; Fiber: 4g; Protein: 7g

Zucchini-Eggplant Gratin

SERVES

6

PREP TIME

10

COOK TIME

20

When those summer vegetables are finally available in abundance in your local store, at farmers' markets, or, if you're lucky, from a home garden, make this veggie entrée. When she has the time, Deanna slices the zucchini and eggplant into thin slices, which layer into a beautiful dish, but that method adds a lot of pan-frying time. Here, she sped up the process by finely chopping the veggies so you can get your gratin on the table in a half hour.

1 large eggplant, finely chopped (about 5 cups)

2 large zucchini, finely chopped (about 3¾ cups)

¼ teaspoon freshly ground black pepper

¼ teaspoon kosher or sea salt

3 tablespoons extra-virgin olive oil, divided

1 tablespoon all-purpose flour

¾ cup 2% milk

⅓ cup plus 2 tablespoons grated Parmesan cheese, divided

1 cup chopped tomato (about 1 large tomato)

1 cup diced or shredded fresh mozzarella (about 4 ounces)

¼ cup fresh basil leaves

1. Preheat the oven to 425°F.

2. In a large bowl, toss together the eggplant, zucchini, pepper, and salt.

3. In a large skillet over medium-high heat, heat 1 tablespoon of oil. Add half the veggie mixture to the skillet. Stir a few times, then cover and cook for 5 minutes, stirring occasionally. Pour the cooked veggies into a baking dish. Place the skillet back on the heat, add 1 tablespoon of oil, and repeat with the remaining veggies. Add the veggies to the baking dish.

4. While the vegetables are cooking, heat the milk in the microwave for 1 minute. Set aside.

5. Place a medium saucepan over medium heat. Add the remaining tablespoon of oil and flour, and whisk together for about 1 minute, until well blended.

6. Slowly pour the warm milk into the oil mixture, whisking the entire time. Continue to whisk frequently until the mixture thickens a bit. Add ⅓ cup of Parmesan cheese, and whisk until melted. Pour the cheese sauce over the vegetables in the baking dish and mix well.

7. Gently mix in the tomatoes and mozzarella cheese. Roast in the oven for 10 minutes, or until the gratin is almost set and not runny. Garnish with the fresh basil leaves and the remaining 2 tablespoons of Parmesan cheese before serving.

Ingredient tip: In the winter months, you can swap in root vegetables for the zucchini and eggplant. Try potatoes, sweet potatoes, beets, turnips, and carrots; double the cooking time both in the skillet and in the oven, as these veggies have much thicker flesh and take longer to cook all the way through.

Per Serving Calories: 207; Total Fat: 14g; Saturated Fat: 5g; Cholesterol: 24mg; Sodium: 311mg; Total Carbohydrates: 12g; Fiber: 4g; Protein: 11g

Grilled Stuffed Portabello Mushrooms

SERVES

6

PREP
TIME

5

COOK
TIME

25

NUT-FREE, GLUTEN-FREE, EGG-FREE, VEGETARIAN

Mushroom lovers, this one's for you. Meaty portabellos replace the traditional pizza crust in these gluten-free "pizzas," proving that vegetarian grilling can be hearty and delicious. Deanna likes making these in the summer, when she has an abundance of summer veggies like tomatoes and zucchini on hand.

3 tablespoons extra-virgin olive oil, divided

1 cup diced onion (about ½ medium onion)

2 garlic cloves, minced (about 1 teaspoon)

3 cups chopped mushrooms, any variety

1 large or 2 small zucchini or summer squash, diced (about 2 cups)

1 cup chopped tomato (about 1 large tomato)

1 teaspoon dried oregano

¼ teaspoon crushed red pepper

¼ teaspoon kosher or sea salt

6 large portabello mushrooms, stems and gills removed

Nonstick cooking spray (if needed)

4 ounces fresh mozzarella cheese, shredded

Additional dried oregano, for serving (optional)

1. In a large skillet over medium heat, heat 2 tablespoons of oil. Add the onion and cook for 4 minutes, stirring occasionally. Stir in the garlic and cook for 1 minute, stirring often.

2. Stir in the mushrooms, zucchini, tomato, oregano, crushed red pepper, and salt. Cook for 10 minutes, stirring occasionally. Remove from the heat.

3. While the veggies are cooking, heat the grill or grill pan to medium-high heat.

4. Brush the remaining tablespoon of oil over the portabello mushroom caps. Place the mushrooms bottom-side (where the stem was removed) down on the grill or pan. Cover and cook for 5 minutes. (If using a grill pan, cover with a sheet of aluminum foil sprayed with nonstick cooking spray.)

5. Flip the mushroom caps over, and spoon about ½ cup of the cooked vegetable mixture into each cap. Top each with about 2½ tablespoons of mozzarella and additional oregano, if desired.

6. Cover and grill for 4 to 5 minutes, or until the cheese melts.

7. Remove each portabello with a spatula, and let them sit for about 5 minutes to cool slightly before serving.

Ingredient tip: Look for large, flat portabello mushroom caps to help make filling them easier. Chop up the stems and add them to the veggie mix before cooking.

Per Serving Calories: 171; Total Fat: 12g; Saturated Fat: 4g; Cholesterol: 15mg; Sodium: 207mg; Total Carbohydrates: 11g; Fiber: 3g; Protein: 9g

Stuffed Tomatoes with Tabbouleh

DAIRY-FREE, EGG-FREE, VEGETARIAN

SERVES

4

PREP TIME

10

COOK TIME

20

Save this recipe for the prime summer tomato season when beefsteak, heirloom, and other round beauties are at their peak. The tabbouleh stuffing is a refreshing salad from the eastern Mediterranean made up of curly parsley, mint, tomatoes, olive oil, lemon juice, and bulgur. Here, we use the quicker-cooking couscous, but feel free to swap in the traditional bulgur—it will take about 15 minutes longer to cook and will use double the water.

8 medium beefsteak or similar tomatoes

3 tablespoons extra-virgin olive oil, divided

½ cup water

½ cup uncooked regular or whole-wheat couscous

1½ cups minced fresh curly parsley (about 1 large bunch)

⅓ cup minced fresh mint

2 scallions, green and white parts, chopped (about 2 tablespoons)

¼ teaspoon freshly ground black pepper

¼ teaspoon kosher or sea salt

1 medium lemon

4 teaspoons honey

⅓ cup chopped almonds

1. Preheat the oven to 400°F.

2. Slice the top off each tomato and set aside. Scoop out all the flesh inside, and put the tops, flesh, and seeds in a large mixing bowl.

3. Grease a baking dish with 1 tablespoon of oil. Place the carved-out tomatoes in the baking dish, and cover with aluminum foil. Roast for 10 minutes.

4. While the tomatoes are cooking, make the couscous by bringing the water to boil in a medium saucepan. Pour in the couscous, remove from the heat, and cover. Let sit for 5 minutes, then stir with a fork.

5. While the couscous is cooking, chop up the tomato flesh and tops. Drain off the excess tomato water using a colander. Measure out 1 cup of the chopped tomatoes (reserve any remaining chopped tomatoes for another use). Add the cup of tomatoes back into the mixing bowl. Mix in the parsley, mint, scallions, pepper, and salt.

6. Using a Microplane or citrus grater, zest the lemon into the mixing bowl. Halve the lemon, and squeeze the juice through a strainer (to catch the seeds) from both halves into the bowl with the tomato mixture. Mix well.

7. When the couscous is ready, add it to the tomato mixture and mix well.

8. With oven mitts, carefully remove the tomatoes from the oven. Divide the tabbouleh evenly among the tomatoes and stuff them, using a spoon to press the filling down so it all fits. Cover the pan with the foil and return it to the oven. Cook for another 8 to 10 minutes, or until the tomatoes are tender-firm. (If you prefer softer tomatoes, roast for an additional 10 minutes.) Before serving, top each tomato with a drizzle of ½ teaspoon of honey and about 2 teaspoons of almonds.

Ingredient tip: Instead of tomatoes, you can use bell peppers and prepare them in the same way. Or halve a zucchini lengthwise, scoop out the seeds, and follow the same instructions. In the fall and winter, try stuffing butternut or acorn squash. Halve the squash and scoop out the seeds. Brush each half with a tablespoon of olive oil and roast for 45 to 60 minutes, or until the squash is cooked through. Stuff with the tabbouleh and serve.

Per Serving Calories: 314; Total Fat: 15g; Saturated Fat: 2g; Cholesterol: 0mg; Sodium: 141mg; Total Carbohydrates: 41g; Fiber: 8g; Protein: 8g

Polenta with Mushroom Bolognese

NUT-FREE, GLUTEN-FREE, EGG-FREE, VEGETARIAN

Serena was able to turn her original Slow Cooker Mushroom Bolognese into a 30-minute version using pantry ingredients like tomato paste, dried oregano, and red wine. Here, we serve it over slices of crispy-fried polenta, but it's also super tasty over thick pasta like ziti, rigatoni, or gnocchi.

2 (8-ounce) packages white button mushrooms

3 tablespoons extra-virgin olive oil, divided

1½ cups finely chopped onion (about ¾ medium onion)

½ cup finely chopped carrot (about 1 medium carrot)

4 garlic cloves, minced (about 2 teaspoons)

1 (18-ounce) tube plain polenta, cut into 8 slices

¼ cup tomato paste

1 tablespoon dried oregano, crushed between your fingers

¼ teaspoon ground nutmeg

¼ teaspoon kosher or sea salt

¼ teaspoon freshly ground black pepper

½ cup dry red wine

½ cup whole milk

½ teaspoon sugar

1. Put half the mushrooms in a food processor bowl and pulse about 15 times until finely chopped but not puréed, similar to the texture of ground meat. Repeat with the remaining mushrooms and set aside. (You can also use the food processor to chop the onion, carrot, and garlic, instead of chopping with a knife.)

2. In a large stockpot over medium-high heat, heat 2 tablespoons of oil. Add the onion and carrot and cook for 5 minutes, stirring occasionally. Add the mushrooms and garlic and cook for 5 minutes, stirring frequently.

3. While the vegetables are cooking, add the remaining 1 tablespoon of oil to a large skillet and heat over medium-high heat. Add 4 slices of polenta to the skillet and cook for 3 to 4 minutes, until golden; flip and cook for 3 to 4 minutes more. Remove the polenta from the skillet, place it on a shallow serving dish, and cover with aluminum foil to keep warm. Repeat with the remaining 4 slices of polenta.

4. To the mushroom mixture in the stockpot, add the tomato paste, oregano, nutmeg, salt, and pepper and stir. Continue cooking for another 2 to 3 minutes, until the vegetables have softened and begun to brown. Add the wine and cook for 1 to 2 minutes, scraping up any bits from the bottom of the pan while stirring with a wooden spoon. Cook until the wine is nearly all evaporated. Lower the heat to medium.

5. Meanwhile, in a small, microwave-safe bowl, mix the milk and sugar together and microwave on high for 30 to 45 seconds, until very hot. Slowly stir the milk into the mushroom mixture and simmer for 4 more minutes, until the milk is absorbed. To serve, pour the mushroom veggie sauce over the warm polenta slices.

Ingredient tip: Don't be surprised by the hefty amount of dried oregano in this dish and other recipes in the book. It's packed with antioxidants, plus that quintessential Italian "pizza" flavor. Serena uses it often in her kitchen, adding it to everything from scrambled eggs to soups. Crumble it between your fingers to release the flavorful oils when adding it to a recipe.

Per Serving Calories: 300; Total Fat: 12g; Saturated Fat: 2g; Cholesterol: 3mg; Sodium: 471mg; Total Carbohydrates: 38g; Fiber: 5g; Protein: 9g

North African Peanut Stew over Cauliflower Rice

GLUTEN-FREE, VEGAN

Our Slow Cooker North African Peanut Stew is one of the most popular recipes on our blog, so we were up to the challenge of making a speedier version for this book. The combo of peppery ginger, earthy cumin, and sweet allspice all comes together in a thick broth made rich and creamy by a surprise ingredient: peanut butter.

1 cup frozen corn

2 tablespoons extra-virgin olive oil

1 cup chopped onion (about ½ medium onion)

2 medium Yukon Gold potatoes, unpeeled, cut into ½-inch cubes (about 2 cups)

1 large sweet potato, unpeeled,cut into ½-inch cubes (about 2 cups)

3 garlic cloves, minced (about 1½ teaspoons)

1½ teaspoons ground cumin

1 teaspoon ground allspice

1 teaspoon freshly grated ginger root or ½ teaspoon ground ginger

½ teaspoon crushed red pepper, or to taste

¼ teaspoon kosher or sea salt

½ cup water

1 (28-ounce) can diced tomatoes, undrained

1 (12-ounce) package frozen plain cauliflower rice

1 (15-ounce) can lentils, undrained

⅓ cup creamy peanut butter

Pickled hot peppers, chopped roasted peanuts, chopped fresh cilantro, for serving (optional)

1. Put the corn on the counter to partially thaw while making the stew.

2. In a large stockpot over medium-high heat, heat the oil. Add the onion, potatoes, and sweet potatoes. Cook for 7 minutes, stirring occasionally, until some of the potatoes and onion get golden and crispy. Move the potatoes to the edges of the pot, and add the garlic, cumin, allspice, ginger, crushed red pepper, and salt. Cook for 1 minute, stirring constantly. Stir in the water and cook for 1 more minute, scraping up the crispy bits from the bottom of the pan.

3. Add the tomatoes with their juices to the stockpot. Cook for 15 minutes uncovered, stirring occasionally.

4. While the tomatoes are cooking, cook the cauliflower rice according to the package directions.

5. Into the tomato mixture, stir in the lentils, partially thawed corn, and peanut butter. Reduce the heat to medium and cook for 1 to 2 minutes, until all the ingredients are warmed, stirring constantly to blend in the peanut butter. Serve over the cauliflower rice with hot peppers, peanuts, and fresh cilantro, if desired.

Prep tip: If you prefer the original set-it-and-forget-it slow cooker recipe, check out TeaspoonOfSpice.com.

Per Serving Calories: 467; Total Fat: 20g; Saturated Fat: 4g; Cholesterol: 0mg; Sodium: 270mg; Total Carbohydrates: 66g; Fiber: 16g; Protein: 21g

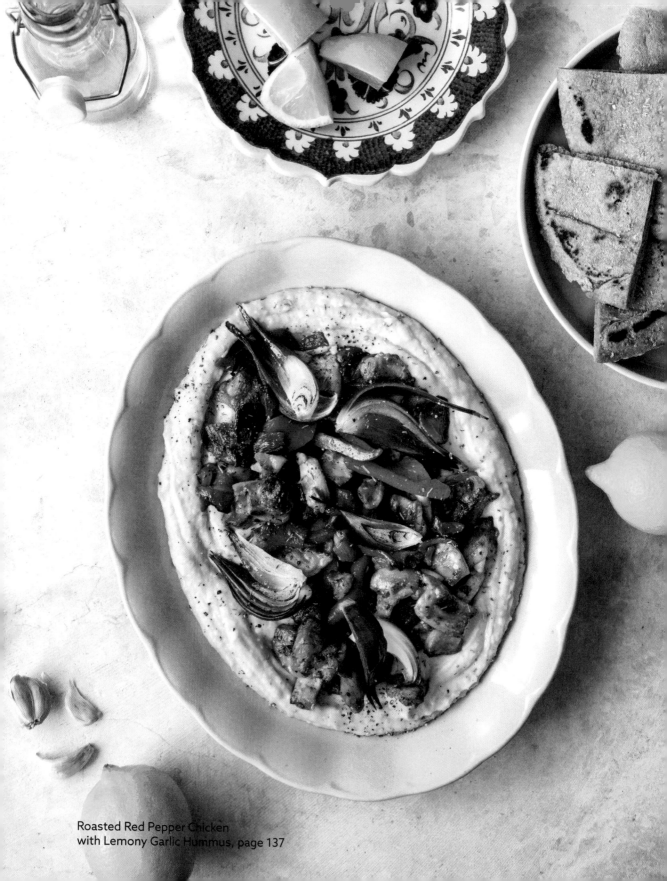

Roasted Red Pepper Chicken
with Lemony Garlic Hummus, page 137

TEN

Chicken

GRILLED, baked, broiled, poached—we're using every cooking trick in the book to deliver 10 terrific chicken meals to you. From finger-licking-good Peach-Glazed Chicken Drummies (page 141) to the comfort of One-Pan Parsley Chicken and Potatoes (page 134), there's a 30-minute-or-less option for everyone's tastes, all with a Mediterranean flair. Feel free to swap in turkey in any of these recipes, as you like.

Grilled Oregano Chicken Kebabs with Zucchini and Olives

SERVES

4

PREP TIME

10

COOK TIME

20

DAIRY-FREE, NUT-FREE, GLUTEN-FREE, EGG-FREE, ONE POT

Featuring Mediterranean pantry staples, these kebabs are a quick-fix dinner to whip up on a busy weeknight, and it's easy enough to double the ingredients when you're having guests over for a barbecue. The recipe includes olive brine—the salty juice the olives are packed in—for extra flavor.

Nonstick cooking spray

¼ cup extra-virgin olive oil

2 tablespoons balsamic vinegar

1 teaspoon dried oregano, crushed between your fingers

1 pound boneless, skinless chicken breasts, cut into 1½-inch pieces

2 medium zucchini, cut into 1-inch pieces (about 2½ cups)

½ cup Kalamata olives, pitted and halved

2 tablespoons olive brine

¼ cup torn fresh basil leaves

Per Serving Calories: 264; Total Fat: 16g; Saturated Fat: 2g; Cholesterol: 65mg; Sodium: 209mg; Total Carbohydrates: 5g; Fiber: 2g; Protein: 27g

1. Coat the cold grill with nonstick cooking spray. Heat the grill to medium-high.

2. In a small bowl, whisk together the oil, vinegar, and oregano. Divide the marinade between two large plastic zip-top bags.

3. Add the chicken to one bag and the zucchini to another. Seal and massage the marinade into both the chicken and zucchini.

4. Thread the chicken onto 6 (12-inch) wooden skewers. Thread the zucchini onto 8 or 9 (12-inch) wooden skewers. Cook the kebabs in batches on the grill for 5 minutes, flip, and grill for 5 minutes more, until any chicken juices run clear.

5. Remove the chicken and zucchini from the skewers and put in a large serving bowl. Toss with the olives, olive brine, and basil and serve.

Prep tip: You can also make this dish without the skewers in a large skillet or grill pan on the stove top. Cook the chicken pieces for about 8 minutes, or until the internal temperature of the chicken is 165°F on a meat thermometer and any juices run clear, stirring occasionally. Remove from the skillet, then cook the zucchini for 8 to 10 minutes, or until softened, stirring occasionally. Toss the chicken, zucchini, and remaining ingredients together in a large serving bowl.

Honey Almond–Crusted Chicken Tenders

~~~~~~~~~~~~~~~~~~~~~~~~~~~~~~~~

DAIRY-FREE, GLUTEN-FREE, EGG-FREE, 5 INGREDIENTS, ONE POT

~~~~~~~~~~~~~~~~~~~~~~~~~~~~~~~~

Here we take pieces of chicken breast tenders, dip them in a finger lickin' sticky-sweet sauce, encase them in crunchy almonds, and then bake. Eat them with a knife and fork—or with your fingers, like the kids—and pair them with a tasty side salad or the filling from our Greek Salad Wraps (page 76).

Nonstick cooking spray

1 tablespoon honey

1 tablespoon whole-grain or Dijon mustard

¼ teaspoon kosher or sea salt

¼ teaspoon freshly ground black pepper

1 pound boneless, skinless chicken breast tenders or tenderloins

1 cup almonds (about 3 ounces)

Per Serving Calories: 263; Total Fat: 12g; Saturated Fat: 1g; Cholesterol: 65mg; Sodium: 237mg; Total Carbohydrates: 9g; Fiber: 3g; Protein: 31g

1. Preheat the oven to 425°F. Line a large, rimmed baking sheet with parchment paper. Place a wire cooling rack on the parchment-lined baking sheet, and coat the rack well with nonstick cooking spray.

2. In a large bowl, combine the honey, mustard, salt, and pepper. Add the chicken and stir gently to coat. Set aside.

3. Use a knife or a mini food processor to roughly chop the almonds; they should be about the size of sunflower seeds. Dump the nuts onto a large sheet of parchment paper and spread them out. Press the coated chicken tenders into the nuts until evenly coated on all sides. Place the chicken on the prepared wire rack.

4. Bake for 15 to 20 minutes, or until the internal temperature of the chicken measures 165°F on a meat thermometer and any juices run clear. Serve immediately.

Prep tip: We like to use parchment paper to make lots of kitchen tasks easier. Often we line our baking sheets with it to make cleanup a snap after cooking. And to keep parchment paper from rolling up when lining a baking sheet: Scrunch it into a ball, then flatten it out; it will stay smooth and flat.

One-Pan Parsley Chicken and Potatoes

SERVES

6

PREP
TIME

5

COOK
TIME

25

DAIRY-FREE, NUT-FREE, GLUTEN-FREE, EGG-FREE, ONE POT

This soul-satisfying skillet of chicken and potatoes is inspired by the sunny South of France, which lies on the Mediterranean Sea. Simple ingredients like lemon, parsley, and Dijon mustard flavor this dish into something to make you smile. It made Serena's kids especially happy; it's their highest rated recipe in this book!

1½ pounds boneless, skinless chicken thighs, cut into 1-inch cubes

1 tablespoon extra-virgin olive oil

1½ pounds Yukon Gold potatoes, unpeeled, cut into ½-inch cubes (about 6 small potatoes)

2 garlic cloves, minced (about 1 teaspoon)

¼ cup dry white wine or apple cider vinegar

1 cup low-sodium or no-salt-added chicken broth

1 tablespoon Dijon mustard

¼ teaspoon kosher or sea salt

¼ teaspoon freshly ground black pepper

1 cup chopped fresh flat-leaf (Italian) parsley, including stems

1 tablespoon freshly squeezed lemon juice (½ small lemon)

1. Pat the chicken dry with a few paper towels. In a large skillet over medium-high heat, heat the oil. Add the chicken and cook for 5 minutes, stirring only after the chicken has browned on one side. Remove the chicken from the pan with a slotted spoon, and put it on a plate; it will not yet be fully cooked. Leave the skillet on the stove.

2. Add the potatoes to the skillet and cook for 5 minutes, stirring only after the potatoes have become golden and crispy on one side. Push the potatoes to the side of the skillet, add the garlic, and cook, stirring constantly, for 1 minute. Add the wine and cook for 1 minute, until nearly evaporated. Add the chicken broth, mustard, salt, pepper, and reserved chicken pieces. Turn the heat up to high, and bring to a boil.

3. Once boiling, cover the skillet, reduce the heat to medium-low, and cook for 10 to 12 minutes, until the potatoes are tender and the internal temperature of the chicken measures 165°F on a meat thermometer and any juices run clear.

4. During the last minute of cooking, stir in the parsley. Remove from the heat, stir in the lemon juice, and serve.

Prep tip: You may wonder why we ask that you pat the chicken dry (or pat the meat dry in the Turkish Lamb Stew, page 160). Without a dry surface on your poultry or meat, it won't get a nicely browned crust.

Per Serving Calories: 241; Total Fat: 4g; Saturated Fat: 1g; Cholesterol: 65mg; Sodium: 245mg; Total Carbohydrates: 20g; Fiber: 3g; Protein: 29g

Romesco Poached Chicken

SERVES

6

PREP TIME

5

COOK TIME

20

Another reason we love our Romesco Dip (page 32) is that it makes an incredible topping, both in flavor and presentation, when served with meat, fish, vegetables, and here, chicken. You can use chicken thighs in this recipe if you'd like, but check the internal temperature a few minutes sooner than you would when cooking chicken breasts.

1½ pounds boneless, skinless chicken breasts, cut into 6 pieces

1 carrot, halved

1 celery stalk, halved

½ onion, halved

2 garlic cloves, smashed

3 sprigs fresh thyme or rosemary

1 cup Romesco Dip (page 32)

2 tablespoons chopped fresh flat-leaf (Italian) parsley

¼ teaspoon freshly ground black pepper

1. Put the chicken in a medium saucepan. Fill with water until there's about one inch of liquid above the chicken. Add the carrot, celery, onion, garlic, and thyme. Cover and bring it to a boil. Reduce the heat to low (keeping it covered), and cook for 12 to 15 minutes, or until the internal temperature of the chicken measures 165°F on a meat thermometer and any juices run clear.

2. Remove the chicken from the water and let sit for 5 minutes.

3. When you're ready to serve, spread ¾ cup of romesco dip on the bottom of a serving platter. Arrange the chicken breasts on top, and drizzle with the remaining romesco dip. Sprinkle the tops with parsley and pepper.

Per Serving Calories: 237; Total Fat: 11g; Saturated Fat: 1g; Cholesterol: 65mg; Sodium: 336mg; Total Carbohydrates: 8g; Fiber: 4g; Protein: 28g

Prep tip: Poaching chicken breasts or thighs is a foolproof way to ensure juicy, moist chicken. Deanna likes to use this method for her Pastina Chicken Soup with Kale (page 47.) You can use the leftover cooking liquid as a homemade chicken broth after removing the vegetables with a strainer.

Roasted Red Pepper Chicken with Lemony Garlic Hummus

SERVES

PREP TIME

COOK TIME

The broiler is your best friend when it comes to cooking this chicken fast while adding amazing flavor with a blast of smoky heat. The result is morsels of char-broiled chicken, onions, and peppers served on a platter of hummus with pita bread for scooping.

1¼ pounds boneless, skinless chicken thighs, cut into 1-inch pieces

½ sweet or red onion, cut into 1-inch chunks (about 1 cup)

2 tablespoons extra-virgin olive oil

½ teaspoon dried thyme

¼ teaspoon freshly ground black pepper

¼ teaspoon kosher or sea salt

1 (12-ounce) jar roasted red peppers, drained and chopped

Lemony Garlic Hummus (page 31), or a 10-ounce container prepared hummus

½ medium lemon

3 (6-inch) whole-wheat pita breads, cut into eighths

1. Line a large, rimmed baking sheet with aluminum foil. Set aside. Set one oven rack about 4 inches below the broiler element. Preheat the broiler to high.

2. In a large bowl, mix together the chicken, onion, oil, thyme, pepper, and salt. Spread the mixture onto the prepared baking sheet.

3. Place the chicken under the broiler and broil for 5 minutes. Remove the pan, stir in the red peppers, and return to the broiler. Broil for another 5 minutes, or until the chicken and onion just start to char on the tips. Remove from the oven.

4. Spread the hummus onto a large serving platter, and spoon the chicken mixture on top. Squeeze the juice from half a lemon over the top, and serve with the pita pieces.

Ingredient tip: Swap in shrimp, salmon, or cod to make this a broiled seafood meal instead. You could also use mushrooms or zucchini as the vegetables, but keep an eye on them, as they will cook faster than the onion.

Per Serving Calories: 324; Total Fat: 11g; Saturated Fat: 2g; Cholesterol: 54mg; Sodium: 625mg; Total Carbohydrates: 29g; Fiber: 6g; Protein: 29g

Tahini Chicken Rice Bowls

NUT-FREE, GLUTEN-FREE, EGG-FREE, ONE POT

Here's our Mediterranean take on popular rice bowls, featuring the seductive flavors of toasty tahini, dried apricots, smoky cumin, and sweet cinnamon. We layer everything side by side in each individual bowl, but you can also mix everything together in a large serving dish for a no-fuss presentation.

SERVES

4

PREP TIME

10

COOK TIME

15

1 cup uncooked instant brown rice

¼ cup tahini or peanut butter (tahini for nut-free)

¼ cup 2% plain Greek yogurt

2 tablespoons chopped scallions, green and white parts (2 scallions)

1 tablespoon freshly squeezed lemon juice (from ½ medium lemon)

1 tablespoon water

1 teaspoon ground cumin

¾ teaspoon ground cinnamon

¼ teaspoon kosher or sea salt

2 cups chopped cooked chicken breast (about 1 pound)

½ cup chopped dried apricots

2 cups peeled and chopped seedless cucumber (1 large cucumber)

4 teaspoons sesame seeds

Fresh mint leaves, for serving (optional)

1. Cook the brown rice according to the package instructions.

2. While the rice is cooking, in a medium bowl, mix together the tahini, yogurt, scallions, lemon juice, water, cumin, cinnamon, and salt. Transfer half the tahini mixture to another medium bowl. Mix the chicken into the first bowl.

3. When the rice is done, mix it into the second bowl of tahini (the one without the chicken).

4. To assemble, divide the chicken among four bowls. Spoon the rice mixture next to the chicken in each bowl. Next to the chicken, place the dried apricots, and in the remaining empty section, add the cucumbers. Sprinkle with sesame seeds, and top with mint, if desired, and serve.

Ingredient tip: Tahini is a paste made from toasted ground sesame seeds, with a consistency similar to peanut butter. It's a staple in eastern Mediterranean dishes like hummus, dips for bread, and desserts. Store it in the refrigerator to keep the sesame oil fresh, and try it in our Beef Gyros with Tahini Sauce (page 152.)

Per Serving Calories: 420; Total Fat: 13g; Saturated Fat: 2g; Cholesterol: 55mg; Sodium: 191mg; Total Carbohydrates: 46g; Fiber: 5g; Protein: 29g

Sheet Pan Lemon Chicken and Roasted Artichokes

DAIRY-FREE, NUT-FREE, GLUTEN-FREE, EGG-FREE, 5 INGREDIENTS, ONE POT

SERVES

4

PREP
TIME

10

COOK
TIME

20

Rarely do just five ingredients come together to make such a flavorful (and impressive) meal. If you've never cooked fresh artichokes, this method of roasting is by far the easiest way. And while Serena's family won't eat every veggie, these lemony roasted artichokes have become a requested favorite.

2 large lemons

3 tablespoons extra-virgin olive oil, divided

½ teaspoon kosher or sea salt

2 large artichokes

4 (6-ounce) bone-in, skin-on chicken thighs

1. Put a large, rimmed baking sheet in the oven. Preheat the oven to 450°F with the pan inside. Tear off four sheets of aluminum foil about 8-by-10 inches each; set aside.

2. Using a Microplane or citrus zester, zest 1 lemon into a large bowl. Halve both lemons and squeeze all the juice into the bowl with the zest. Whisk in 2 tablespoons of oil and the salt. Set aside.

3. Rinse the artichokes with cool water, and dry with a clean towel. Using a sharp knife, cut about 1½ inches off the tip of each artichoke. Cut about ¼ inch off each stem. Halve each artichoke lengthwise so each piece has equal amounts of stem. Immediately plunge the artichoke halves into the lemon juice and oil mixture (to prevent browning) and turn to coat on all sides. Lay one artichoke half flat-side down in the center of a sheet of aluminum foil, and close up loosely to make a foil packet. Repeat the process with the remaining three artichoke halves. Set the packets aside.

CONTINUES NEXT PAGE

4. Put the chicken in the remaining lemon juice mixture and turn to coat.

5. Using oven mitts, carefully remove the hot baking sheet from the oven and pour on the remaining tablespoon of oil; tilt the pan to coat. Carefully arrange the chicken, skin-side down, on the hot baking sheet. Place the artichoke packets, flat-side down, on the baking sheet as well. (Arrange the artichoke packets and chicken with space between them so air can circulate around them.)

6. Roast for 20 minutes, or until the internal temperature of the chicken measures 165°F on a meat thermometer and any juices run clear. Before serving, check the artichokes for doneness by pulling on a leaf. If it comes out easily, the artichoke is ready.

Ingredient tip: Artichokes turn brown *very* quickly after slicing when exposed to air; however, they will still be a beautiful golden color after roasting, and their flavor will not be affected. If artichokes are not in season, use 8 to 12 frozen artichoke hearts instead (no need to thaw).

Per Serving Calories: 372; Total Fat: 29g; Saturated Fat: 8g; Cholesterol: 98mg; Sodium: 381mg; Total Carbohydrates: 11g; Fiber: 5g; Protein: 20g

Peach-Glazed Chicken Drummies

DAIRY-FREE, NUT-FREE, GLUTEN-FREE, EGG-FREE

SERVES

4

PREP
TIME

10

COOK
TIME

20

Satisfy your craving for sticky, drippy, kickin' barbecue chicken with our Mediterranean-style sweet and smoky glaze. This thick and fruity sauce is also terrific on pork, fish, beef, or even grilled veggies.

8 chicken drumsticks
(about 2 pounds),
skin removed

Nonstick cooking spray

1 (15-ounce) can sliced
peaches in 100%
juice, drained

¼ cup honey

¼ cup cider vinegar

3 garlic cloves

½ teaspoon
smoked paprika

¼ teaspoon kosher
or sea salt

¼ teaspoon freshly
ground black pepper

1. Remove the chicken from the refrigerator.

2. Set one oven rack about 4 inches below the broiler element. Preheat the oven to 500°F. Line a large, rimmed baking sheet with aluminum foil. Place a wire cooling rack on the aluminum foil, and spray the rack with nonstick cooking spray. Set aside.

3. In a blender, combine the peaches, honey, vinegar, garlic, smoked paprika, salt, and pepper. Purée the ingredients until smooth.

4. Add the purée to a medium saucepan and bring to a boil over medium-high heat. Cook for 2 minutes, stirring constantly. Divide the sauce among two small bowls. The first bowl will be brushed on the chicken; set aside the second bowl for serving at the table.

CONTINUES NEXT PAGE

5. Brush all sides of the chicken with about half the sauce (keeping half the sauce for a second coating), and place the drumsticks on the prepared rack. Roast for 10 minutes.

6. Remove the chicken from the oven and turn to the high broiler setting. Brush the chicken with the remaining sauce from the first bowl. Return the chicken to the oven and broil for 5 minutes. Turn the chicken; broil for 3 to 5 more minutes, until the internal temperature measures 165°F on a meat thermometer, or until the juices run clear. Serve with the reserved sauce.

Ingredient tip: Fruit canned in 100 percent juice is the perfect ingredient to add natural sweetness to this sauce, instead of the brown sugar or molasses used in many barbecue recipes. Feel free to substitute canned apricots, pears, or even pineapple for the peaches in this recipe.

Per Serving Calories: 291; Total Fat: 5g; Saturated Fat: 1g; Cholesterol: 100mg; Sodium: 224mg; Total Carbohydrates: 33g; Fiber: 2g; Protein: 30g

Baked Chicken Caprese

NUT-FREE, GLUTEN-FREE, EGG-FREE

Featuring the colors of the Italian flag (red tomato, white mozzarella, and green basil), this dish is the answer when you need a no-fuss, weeknight chicken dinner. It's equally good when made on the grill—the chicken will cook up even faster this way.

Nonstick cooking spray

1 pound boneless, skinless chicken breasts

2 tablespoons extra-virgin olive oil

¼ teaspoon freshly ground black pepper

¼ teaspoon kosher or sea salt

1 large tomato, sliced thinly

1 cup shredded mozzarella or 4 ounces fresh mozzarella cheese, diced

1 (14.5-ounce) can low-sodium or no-salt-added crushed tomatoes

2 tablespoons fresh torn basil leaves

4 teaspoons balsamic vinegar

1. Set one oven rack about 4 inches below the broiler element. Preheat the oven to 450°F. Line a large, rimmed baking sheet with aluminum foil. Place a wire cooling rack on the aluminum foil, and spray the rack with nonstick cooking spray. Set aside.

2. Cut the chicken into 4 pieces (if they aren't already). Put the chicken breasts in a large zip-top plastic bag. With a rolling pin or meat mallet, pound the chicken so it is evenly flattened, about ¼-inch thick. Add the oil, pepper, and salt to the bag. Reseal the bag, and massage the ingredients into the chicken. Take the chicken out of the bag and place it on the prepared wire rack.

3. Cook the chicken for 15 to 18 minutes, or until the internal temperature of the chicken is 165°F on a meat thermometer and the juices run clear. Turn the oven to the high broiler setting. Layer the tomato slices on each chicken breast, and top with the mozzarella. Broil the chicken for another 2 to 3 minutes, or until the cheese is melted (don't let the chicken burn on the edges). Remove the chicken from the oven.

CONTINUES NEXT PAGE

4. While the chicken is cooking, pour the crushed tomatoes into a small, microwave-safe bowl. Cover the bowl with a paper towel, and microwave for about 1 minute on high, until hot. When you're ready to serve, divide the tomatoes among four dinner plates. Place each chicken breast on top of the tomatoes. Top with the basil and a drizzle of balsamic vinegar.

Prep tip: Fresh basil and mint leaves are very delicate, so treat them gently when cooking with them. Wait until right before you need them to cut or tear them, as they bruise easily and will turn brown soon after they are cut. Use these herbs interchangeably in recipes.

Per Serving Calories: 312; Total Fat: 15g; Saturated Fat: 1g; Cholesterol: 85mg; Sodium: 412mg; Total Carbohydrates: 11g; Fiber: 4g; Protein: 34g

Grape Chicken Panzanella

EGG-FREE, ONE POT, HALF THE TIME

Upgrade your basic chicken salad to this flavorful twist on the Italian panzanella bread salad. It's studded with sweet grapes, juicy tomatoes, buttery walnuts, creamy Gorgonzola, and tangy red onions.

SERVES

6

PREP TIME

10

COOK TIME

5

3 cups day-old bread (like a baguette, crusty Italian bread, or whole-grain bread), cut into 1-inch cubes

5 tablespoons extra-virgin olive oil, divided

2 cups chopped cooked chicken breast (about 1 pound)

1 cup red seedless grapes, halved

½ pint grape or cherry tomatoes, halved (about ¾ cup)

½ cup Gorgonzola cheese crumbles (about 2 ounces)

1/3 cup chopped walnuts

¼ cup diced red onion (about ⅛ onion)

3 tablespoons chopped fresh mint leaves

¼ teaspoon freshly ground black pepper

1 tablespoon balsamic vinegar

Zest and juice of 1 small lemon

1 teaspoon honey

1. Line a large, rimmed baking sheet with aluminum foil. Set aside. Set one oven rack about 4 inches below the broiler element. Preheat the broiler to high.

2. In a large serving bowl, drizzle the cubed bread with 2 tablespoons of oil, and mix gently with your hands to coat. Spread the mixture over the prepared baking sheet. Place the baking sheet under the broiler for 2 minutes. Stir the bread, then broil for another 30 to 60 seconds, watching carefully so the bread pieces are toasted and not burned. Remove from the oven and set aside.

3. In the same (now empty) large serving bowl, mix together the chicken, grapes, tomatoes, Gorgonzola, walnuts, onion, mint, and pepper. Add the toasted bread pieces, and gently mix together.

4. In a small bowl, whisk together the remaining 3 tablespoons of oil, vinegar, zest and juice from the lemon, and honey. Drizzle the dressing over the salad, toss gently to mix, and serve.

Prep tip: Pack this panzanella salad for lunch in a mason jar. Layer all the ingredients starting with the dressing and the chicken on the bottom and ending with the bread on top. When you're ready to eat, just shake the jar well.

Per Serving Calories:380; Total Fat: 21g; Saturated Fat: 5g; Cholesterol: 64mg; Sodium: 291mg; Total Carbohydrates: 23g

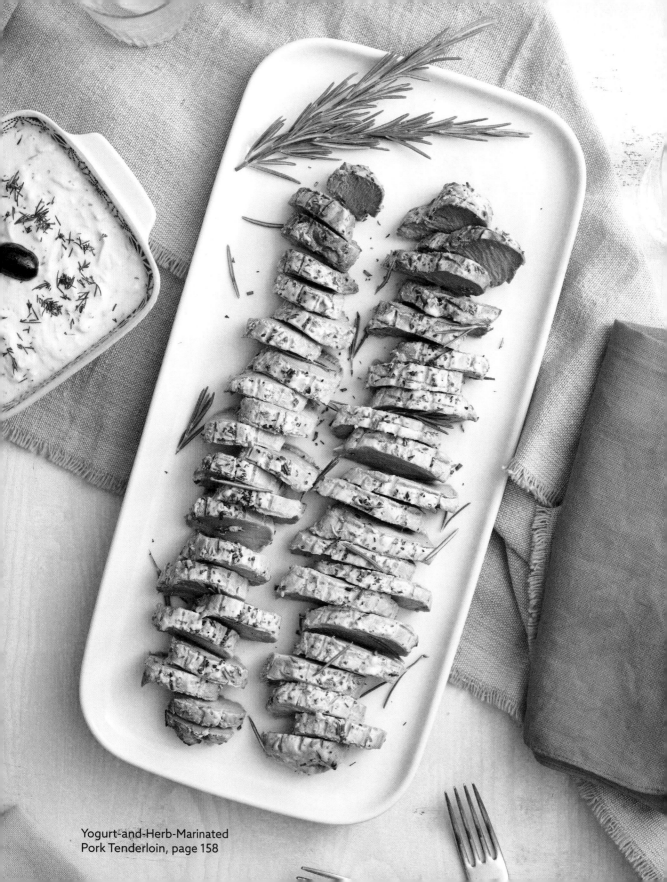

Yogurt-and-Herb-Marinated
Pork Tenderloin, page 158

ELEVEN

Meat

THE Mediterranean Diet features meat more as a side dish than as the main attraction on your dinner plate, so we've used this philosophy to bring you the beef, pork, and lamb dishes you crave, but in a better-for-you fashion. These dishes are just as hearty and mouthwatering but are portioned more reasonably and paired with the vegetables, grains, beans, herbs, and spices that you've seen throughout this cookbook. Get ready for Beef Gyros with Tahini Sauce (page 152), Moroccan Meatballs (page 148), and more!

Moroccan Meatballs

DAIRY-FREE, NUT-FREE, ONE POT

At Serena's house, the resounding cry is, "Yay, meatballs for dinner!" This recipe features ingredients you don't typically see in meatballs—like raisins, cumin, and cinnamon—but the spicy, slightly sweet results are worth savoring. Serve them over brown rice along with the flavorful sauce.

PREP
TIME

10

COOK
TIME

20

¼ cup finely chopped onion (about ⅛ onion)

¼ cup raisins, coarsely chopped

1 teaspoon ground cumin

½ teaspoon ground cinnamon

¼ teaspoon smoked paprika

1 large egg

1 pound ground beef (93% lean) or ground lamb

⅓ cup panko bread crumbs

1 teaspoon extra-virgin olive oil

1 (28-ounce) can low-sodium or no-salt-added crushed tomatoes

Chopped fresh mint, feta cheese, and/or fresh orange or lemon wedges, for serving (optional)

Per Serving Calories: 306; Total Fat: 10g; Saturated Fat: 4g; Cholesterol: 117mg; Sodium: 342mg; Total Carbohydrates: 26g; Fiber: 7g; Protein: 29g

1. In a large bowl, combine the onion, raisins, cumin, cinnamon, smoked paprika, and egg. Add the ground beef and bread crumbs and mix gently with your hands. Divide the mixture into 20 even portions, then wet your hands and roll each portion into a ball. Wash your hands.

2. In a large skillet over medium-high heat, heat the oil. Add the meatballs and cook for 8 minutes, rolling around every minute or so with tongs or a fork to brown them on most sides. (They won't be cooked through.) Transfer the meatballs to a paper towel–lined plate. Drain the fat out of the pan, and carefully wipe out the hot pan with a paper towel.

3. Return the meatballs to the pan, and pour the tomatoes over the meatballs. Cover and cook on medium-high heat until the sauce begins to bubble. Lower the heat to medium, cover partially, and cook for 7 to 8 more minutes, until the meatballs are cooked through. Garnish with fresh mint, feta cheese, and/or a squeeze of citrus, if desired, and serve.

Prep tip: If you have a cast iron skillet, this is the time to pull it out—it's Serena's skillet of choice. Because cast iron holds heat very well, the skillet will cook all 20 meatballs more evenly at the same time. If you don't have a cast iron skillet, add about 3 to 5 minutes to the cooking time in step 2.

Beef Spanakopita Pita Pockets

EGG-FREE, ONE POT

Here we've taken the classic ingredients of Greek spanakopita—spinach and feta—and combined them with lean ground beef, ricotta cheese, and almonds to make a yummy, quick, skillet-cooked filling for whole-wheat pita bread. Yes, the amount of spinach listed is correct—it cooks down to a much smaller amount.

3 teaspoons extra-virgin olive oil, divided

1 pound ground beef (93% lean)

2 garlic cloves, minced (about 1 teaspoon)

2 (6-ounce) bags baby spinach, chopped (about 12 cups)

½ cup crumbled feta cheese (about 2 ounces)

⅓ cup ricotta cheese

½ teaspoon ground nutmeg

¼ teaspoon freshly ground black pepper

¼ cup slivered almonds

4 (6-inch) whole-wheat pita breads, cut in half

Per Serving Calories: 506; Total Fat: 22g; Saturated Fat: 8g; Cholesterol: 98mg; Sodium: 567mg; Total Carbohydrates: 42g; Fiber: 8g; Protein: 39g

1. In a large skillet over medium heat, heat 1 teaspoon of oil. Add the ground beef and cook for 10 minutes, breaking it up with a wooden spoon and stirring occasionally. Remove from the heat and drain in a colander. Set the meat aside.

2. Place the skillet back on the heat, and add the remaining 2 teaspoons of oil. Add the garlic and cook for 1 minute, stirring constantly. Add the spinach and cook for 2 to 3 minutes, or until the spinach has cooked down, stirring often.

3. Turn off the heat and mix in the feta cheese, ricotta, nutmeg, and pepper. Stir until all the ingredients are well incorporated. Mix in the almonds.

4. Divide the beef filling among the eight pita pocket halves to stuff them and serve.

Ingredient tip: You can also use a 10-ounce package of frozen spinach in place of the two bags of fresh spinach. Thaw and cook according to the package instructions, then place in a dish towel. Wrap and squeeze it over the sink to remove as much liquid as possible. Add the cooked spinach to the skillet, heat up for 1 minute, then follow step 3.

Grilled Steak, Mushroom, and Onion Kebabs

SERVES

4

PREP TIME

10

COOK TIME

10

When Serena makes this recipe, her friends always ask, "What's in this yummy marinade?" It's actually a garlic and rosemary-infused dressing you heat on the grill while the kebabs are cooking, so you can avoid the typical hours of marinating. And to make slicing a raw piece of meat easier—especially if you need very thin slices—freeze it (for no more than 10 minutes) first. This will firm up the meat so a knife slides through it with ease.

Nonstick cooking spray

4 garlic cloves, peeled

2 fresh rosemary sprigs (about 3 inches each)

2 tablespoons extra-virgin olive oil, divided

1 pound boneless top sirloin steak, about 1 inch thick

1 (8-ounce) package white button mushrooms

1 medium red onion, cut into 12 thin wedges

¼ teaspoon coarsely ground black pepper

2 tablespoons red wine vinegar

¼ teaspoon kosher or sea salt

1. Soak 12 (10-inch) wooden skewers in water. Spray the cold grill with nonstick cooking spray, and heat the grill to medium-high.

2. Cut a piece of aluminum foil into a 10-inch square. Place the garlic and rosemary sprigs in the center, drizzle with 1 tablespoon of oil, and wrap tightly to form a foil packet. Place it on the grill, and close the grill cover.

3. Cut the steak into 1-inch cubes. Thread the beef onto the wet skewers, alternating with whole mushrooms and onion wedges. Spray the kebabs thoroughly with nonstick cooking spray, and sprinkle with pepper.

4. Cook the kebabs on the covered grill for 4 to 5 minutes. Turn and grill 4 to 5 more minutes, covered, until a meat thermometer inserted in the meat registers 145°F (medium rare) or 160°F (medium).

5. Remove the foil packet from the grill, open, and, using tongs, place the garlic and rosemary sprigs in a small bowl. Carefully strip the rosemary sprigs of their leaves into the bowl and pour in any accumulated juices and oil from the foil packet. Add the remaining 1 tablespoon of oil and the vinegar and salt. Mash the garlic with a fork, and mix all ingredients in the bowl together. Pour over the finished steak kebabs and serve.

Prep tip: You can make this recipe without using the grill. Follow step 2 to prepare the garlic foil packet, then bake it in a 400°F oven for 20 minutes, or until the garlic is soft. To make the kebabs, follow steps 3 and 4 using a grill pan. To cover the grill pan, use a sheet of foil that's been coated with nonstick cooking spray. Follow the rest of the recipe as written.

Per Serving Calories: 300; Total Fat: 14g; Saturated Fat: 4g; Cholesterol: 101mg; Sodium: 196mg; Total Carbohydrates: 6g; Fiber: 1g; Protein: 36g

Beef Gyros with Tahini Sauce

NUT-FREE, EGG-FREE, ONE POT

If you love gyro sandwiches from your local takeout place, you'll adore this version of herb-spiced meat, crisp veggies, and cool yogurt-sesame sauce—all wrapped up in a warm pita. Gyros are traditionally made with lamb, but we found them to be equally mouthwatering when made with steak.

Nonstick cooking spray

2 tablespoons
extra-virgin olive oil

1 tablespoon dried oregano

1¼ teaspoons garlic
powder, divided

1 teaspoon ground cumin

½ teaspoon freshly
ground black pepper

¼ teaspoon kosher
or sea salt

1 pound beef flank steak,
top round steak, or lamb
leg steak, center cut,
about 1 inch thick

1 medium green bell
pepper, halved and seeded

2 tablespoons tahini
or peanut butter
(tahini for nut-free)

1 tablespoon hot
water (if needed)

½ cup 2% plain
Greek yogurt

1 tablespoon freshly
squeezed lemon juice
(about ½ small lemon)

1 cup thinly sliced red
onion (about ½ onion)

4 (6-inch) whole-wheat
pita breads, warmed

1. Set an oven rack about 4 inches below the broiler element. Preheat the oven broiler to high. Line a large, rimmed baking sheet with foil. Place a wire cooling rack on the foil, and spray the rack with nonstick cooking spray. Set aside.

2. In a small bowl, whisk together the oil, oregano, 1 teaspoon of garlic powder, cumin, pepper, and salt. Rub the oil mixture on all sides of the steak, saving 1 teaspoon of the mixture. Place the steak on the prepared rack. Rub the remaining oil mixture on the bell pepper, and place on the rack, cut-side down. Press the pepper with the heel of your hand to flatten.

3. Broil for 5 minutes. Turn the meat and the pepper pieces, and broil for 2 to 5 more minutes, until the pepper is charred and the internal temperature of the meat measures 145°F on a meat thermometer. Put the pepper and steak on a cutting board to rest for 5 minutes.

4. While the meat is broiling, in a small bowl, whisk the tahini until smooth (adding 1 tablespoon of hot water if your tahini is sticky). Add the remaining ¼ teaspoon of garlic powder and the yogurt and lemon juice, and whisk thoroughly.

5. Slice the steak crosswise into ¼-inch-thick strips. Slice the bell pepper into strips. Divide the steak, bell pepper, and onion among the warm pita breads. Drizzle with tahini sauce and serve.

Prep tip: In this recipe, it's important to watch the steak carefully so it doesn't overcook. Check the temperature after you flip it in step 3, and if it's already at around 120°F, broil for only 2 to 3 minutes and check the temperature again.

Per Serving Calories: 497; Total Fat: 21g; Saturated Fat: 5g; Cholesterol: 53mg; Sodium: 548mg; Total Carbohydrates: 45g; Fiber: 7g; Protein: 36g

Beef Sliders with Pepper Slaw

SERVES

4

PREP TIME

10

COOK TIME

10

Get ready to enjoy the juiciest burger you've ever eaten—made with extra-lean ground beef! The secret is not in the sauce—it's the meaty mushrooms we mix in for moisture and rich flavor. Fresh herbs in the pepper slaw topping also bring some Mediterranean flair to these burgers.

Nonstick cooking spray

1 (8-ounce) package white button mushrooms

2 tablespoons extra-virgin olive oil, divided

1 pound ground beef (93% lean)

2 garlic cloves, minced (about 1 teaspoon)

½ teaspoon kosher or sea salt, divided

¼ teaspoon freshly ground black pepper

1 tablespoon balsamic vinegar

2 bell peppers of different colors, sliced into strips

2 tablespoons torn fresh basil or flat-leaf (Italian) parsley

Mini or slider whole-grain rolls, for serving (optional)

1. Set one oven rack about 4 inches below the broiler element. Preheat the oven broiler to high.

2. Line a large, rimmed baking sheet with aluminum foil. Place a wire cooling rack on the aluminum foil, and spray the rack with nonstick cooking spray. Set aside.

3. Put half the mushrooms in the bowl of a food processor and pulse about 15 times, until the mushrooms are finely chopped but not puréed, similar to the texture of ground meat. Repeat with the remaining mushrooms.

4. In a large skillet over medium-high heat, heat 1 tablespoon of oil. Add the mushrooms and cook for 2 to 3 minutes, stirring occasionally, until the mushrooms have cooked down and some of their liquid has evaporated. Remove from the heat.

5. In a large bowl, combine the ground beef with the cooked mushrooms, garlic, ¼ teaspoon of salt, and pepper. Mix gently using your hands. Form the meat into 8 small (½-inch-thick) patties, and place on the prepared rack, making two lines of 4 patties down the center of the pan.

6. Place the pan in the oven so the broiler heating element is directly over as many burgers as possible. Broil for 4 minutes. Flip the burgers and rearrange them so any burgers not getting brown are nearer to the heat source. Broil for 3 to 4 more minutes, or until the internal temperature of the meat is 160°F on a meat thermometer. Watch carefully to prevent burning.

7. While the burgers are cooking, in a large bowl, whisk together the remaining 1 tablespoon of oil, vinegar, and remaining ¼ teaspoon of salt. Add the peppers and basil, and stir gently to coat with the dressing. Serve the sliders with the pepper slaw as a topping or on the side. If desired, serve with the rolls, burger style.

Prep tip: Blending chopped mushrooms into ground meat is a way to add some veggies and bulk up the size of the burger—or even replace some of the meat. This mushroom-meat blend can be used in any meat-based recipes, including tacos, meatloaf, lasagna, pasta sauce, meatballs, and more.

Per Serving Calories: 259; Total Fat: 15g; Saturated Fat: 4g; Cholesterol: 73mg; Sodium: 315mg; Total Carbohydrates: 5g; Fiber: 2g; Protein: 26g

Mini Greek Meatloaves

SERVES

6

PREP TIME

5

COOK TIME

25

These Greek-style mini meatloaves—stuffed with feta, onion, garlic, and oregano—are baked in a muffin tin so they cook up quickly and are already perfectly portioned. They are topped with a simple yet appealing Kalamata olive yogurt glaze, and Deanna likes to serve them over a bed of lettuce like bunless burgers, or with pieces of pita bread to sop up the extra yummy sauce.

Nonstick cooking spray

1 tablespoon extra-virgin olive oil

½ cup minced onion (about ¼ onion)

1 garlic clove, minced (about ½ teaspoon)

1 pound ground beef (93% lean)

½ cup whole-wheat bread crumbs

½ cup crumbled feta cheese (about 2 ounces)

1 large egg

½ teaspoon dried oregano, crushed between your fingers

¼ teaspoon freshly ground black pepper

½ cup 2% plain Greek yogurt

⅓ cup chopped and pitted Kalamata olives

2 tablespoons olive brine

Romaine lettuce or pita bread, for serving (optional)

1. Preheat the oven to 400°F. Coat a 12-cup muffin pan with nonstick cooking spray and set aside.

2. In a small skillet over medium heat, heat the oil. Add the onion and cook for 4 minutes, stirring frequently. Add the garlic and cook for 1 more minute, stirring frequently. Remove from the heat.

3. In a large mixing bowl, combine the onion and garlic with the ground beef, bread crumbs, feta, egg, oregano, and pepper. Gently mix together with your hands.

4. Divide into 12 portions and place in the muffin cups. Cook for 18 to 20 minutes, or until the internal temperature of the meat is 160°F on a meat thermometer.

5. While the meatloaves are baking, in a small bowl, whisk together the yogurt, olives, and olive brine.

6. When you're ready to serve, place the meatloaves on a serving platter and spoon the olive-yogurt sauce on top. You can also serve them on a bed of lettuce or with cut-up pieces of pita bread.

Prep tip: To make one regular-size meatloaf, use an 8-by-4-inch loaf pan coated with nonstick cooking spray. Cook at 350°F for 35 to 40 minutes, or until the internal temperature of the meat is 160°F. Spoon the yogurt sauce over top, slice, and serve.

Per Serving Calories: 244; Total Fat: 13g; Saturated Fat: 5g; Cholesterol: 87mg; Sodium: 355mg; Total Carbohydrates: 10g; Fiber: 1g; Protein: 22g

Yogurt-and-Herb-Marinated Pork Tenderloin

NUT-FREE, GLUTEN-FREE, EGG-FREE, 5 INGREDIENTS, ONE POT

SERVES

6

PREP TIME

5

COOK TIME

25

Never again will your pork tenderloin be anything but tender, juicy, and perfectly cooked when made with this Mediterranean twist. Tenderloin is a lean cut that's lower in saturated fat, which means it runs the risk of drying out more easily when cooking. Slathering on rosemary-scented yogurt ensures you won't end up with overcooked pork.

Nonstick cooking spray

2 medium pork tenderloins (10 to 12 ounces each)

½ teaspoon freshly ground black pepper

½ teaspoon kosher or sea salt

¼ cup 2% plain Greek yogurt

1 tablespoon chopped fresh rosemary

Tzatziki yogurt sauce from Chickpea Patties in Pitas (page 75, step 3) or store-bought tzatziki sauce

1 to 2 tablespoons chopped fresh mint (optional)

1. Preheat the oven to 500°F.

2. Line a large, rimmed baking sheet with aluminum foil. Place a wire cooling rack on the aluminum foil, and spray the rack with nonstick cooking spray.

3. Place both pieces of the pork on the wire rack, folding under any skinny ends of the meat to ensure even cooking. Sprinkle both pieces evenly with the pepper and salt.

4. In a small bowl, mix together the yogurt and rosemary. Using a spoon or your fingers, slather the yogurt mixture over all sides of the pork.

5. Roast on the wire rack for 10 minutes. Remove the baking sheet from the oven, and turn over both pieces of pork. Roast for 10 to 12 minutes more, or until the internal temperature of the pork measures 145°F on a meat thermometer and the juices run clear. Remove the pork from the rack and place on a clean cutting board. Let rest for 5 minutes, then slice.

6. While the pork is roasting, make the tzatziki yogurt sauce, adding fresh mint to the sauce, if desired. Serve the sauce with the pork.

Prep tip: We cooked several tenderloins and found that two 10.5-ounce tenderloins took a total of exactly 20 minutes to reach 145°F. Two 12-ounce tenderloins took 22 minutes. Plan your cooking time according to these parameters.

Per Serving Calories: 183; Total Fat: 10g; Saturated Fat: 3g; Cholesterol: 73mg; Sodium: 372mg; Total Carbohydrates: 4g; Fiber: 0g; Protein: 22g

Turkish Lamb Stew

SERVES
6

PREP TIME
10

COOK TIME
20

Don't let the long-ish ingredients list or your lack of experience cooking lamb deter you from making this rich, succulent dish. Lamb has been a staple meat in Mediterranean regions for generations, as it pairs well with both sweet and savory flavors—like this stew based on Turkish and Moroccan tagines. Sweet cinnamon and prunes combine with earthy cumin and spicy, smoky peppers in this special meal, which is Serena's husband's favorite recipe in the whole book.

1 pound bone-in or boneless lamb leg steak, center cut

1 tablespoon extra-virgin olive oil

1 cup chopped onion (about ½ onion)

½ cup diced carrot (about 1 medium carrot)

1 teaspoon ground cumin

½ teaspoon ground cinnamon

¼ teaspoon kosher or sea salt

4 garlic cloves, minced (about 2 teaspoons)

2 tablespoons tomato paste

1 tablespoon chopped canned chipotle pepper in adobo sauce

2 cups water

½ cup chopped prunes

1 (15-ounce) can chickpeas, drained and rinsed

2 tablespoons freshly squeezed lemon juice (from 1 small lemon)

¼ cup chopped unsalted pistachios

Cooked couscous or bulgur, for serving (optional)

1. Slice the meat into 1-inch cubes (including the bone-in piece of meat; see the ingredient tip). Pat dry with a few paper towels.

2. In a large stockpot over medium-high heat, heat the oil. Add the lamb and any bone, and cook for 4 minutes, stirring only after allowing the meat to brown on one side. Using a slotted spoon, transfer the lamb from the pot to a plate. It will not yet be fully cooked. Don't clean out the stockpot.

3. Put the onion, carrot, cumin, cinnamon, and salt in the pot and cook for 6 minutes, stirring occasionally. Push the vegetables to the edge of the pot. Add the garlic and cook for 1 minute, stirring constantly. Add the tomato paste and chipotle pepper, and cook for 1 minute more, stirring constantly while blending and mashing the tomato paste into the vegetables.

4. Return the lamb to the pot along with the water and prunes. Turn up the heat to high, and bring to a boil. Reduce the heat to medium-low and cook for 5 to 7 minutes more, until the stew thickens slightly. Stir in the chickpeas and cook for 1 minute. Remove the stew from the heat, and stir in the lemon juice. Sprinkle the pistachios on top and serve over couscous, if desired.

Ingredient tip: Usually lamb leg steak comes with a small round of bone. Add the bone along with the meat to stews or soups for extra rich flavor and for the nutritious minerals that will seep into the gravy.

Per Serving Calories: 509; Total Fat: 17g; Saturated Fat: 5g; Cholesterol: 51mg; Sodium: 299mg; Total Carbohydrates: 29g; Fiber: 5g; Protein: 20g

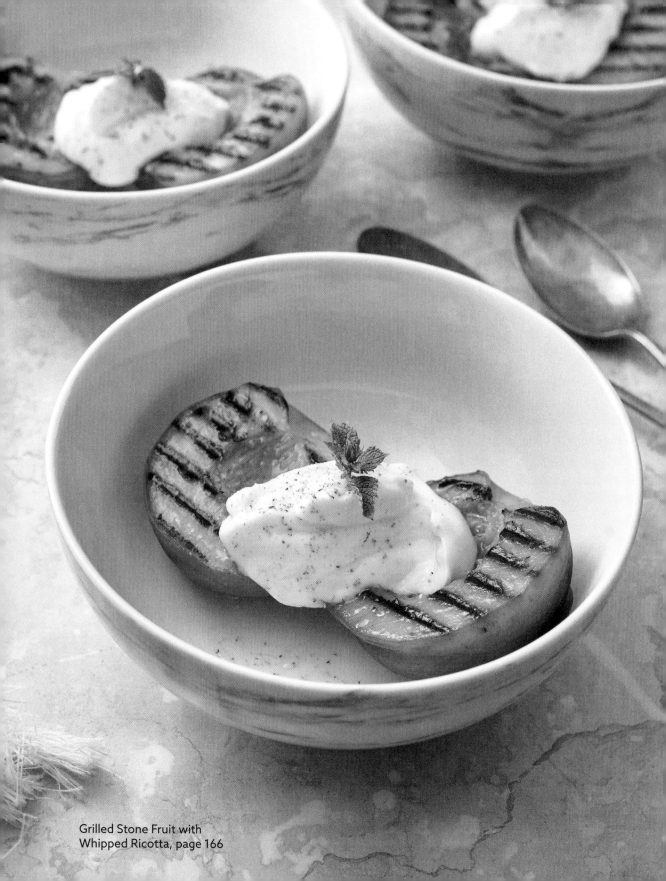

Grilled Stone Fruit with
Whipped Ricotta, page 166

TWELVE

Desserts

WE are dietitians who believe dessert should have a rightful place in any eating lifestyle, especially when the ingredients are simple and the serving sizes are right. From Chilled Dark Chocolate Fruit Kebabs (page 164) to Roasted Orange Rice Pudding (page 171), in this chapter we've relied on Mediterranean staples like honey, fruit, yogurt, and dark chocolate to deliver scrumptious and satisfying sweet endings that won't leave you feeling stuffed.

Chilled Dark Chocolate Fruit Kebabs

SERVES

6

PREP
TIME

10

CHILL
TIME

20

NUT-FREE, GLUTEN-FREE, VEGAN, 5 INGREDIENTS

These five-ingredient dessert skewers are an impressive last-minute option when you want a sweet treat that's fairly low in calories. Make them for those hot summer days when you don't want to heat up the kitchen.

12 strawberries, hulled

12 cherries, pitted

24 seedless red or green grapes

24 blueberries

8 ounces dark chocolate

Per Serving Calories: 254; Total Fat: 15g; Saturated Fat: 8g; Cholesterol: 2mg; Sodium: 5mg; Total Carbohydrates: 29g; Fiber: 4g; Protein: 3g

1. Line a large, rimmed baking sheet with parchment paper. On your work surface, lay out six 12-inch wooden skewers.

2. Thread the fruit onto the skewers, following this pattern: 1 strawberry, 1 cherry, 2 grapes, 2 blueberries, 1 strawberry, 1 cherry, 2 grapes, and 2 blueberries (or vary according to taste!). Place the kebabs on the prepared baking sheet.

3. In a medium, microwave-safe bowl, heat the chocolate in the microwave for 1 minute on high. Stir until the chocolate is completely melted.

4. Spoon the melted chocolate into a small plastic sandwich bag. Twist the bag closed right above the chocolate, and snip the corner of the bag off with scissors. Squeeze the bag to drizzle lines of chocolate over the kebabs.

5. Place the sheet in the freezer and chill for 20 minutes before serving.

Prep tip: Try this with other Mediterranean fruits, like fresh figs, plums, and oranges, or slices of fresh or canned apricots and peaches. You could also use dried figs or prunes.

Vanilla Greek Yogurt Affogato

GLUTEN-FREE, EGG-FREE, VEGETARIAN, 5 INGREDIENTS, HALF THE TIME

SERVES

4

PREP TIME

10

A traditional dessert from Italy, affogato is a shot of espresso poured over ice cream or gelato. Our version uses protein-rich Greek-style yogurt as a better-for-you dessert that still gives that creamy dairy richness but with fewer calories. This recipe calls for vanilla yogurt, but it works well with other flavors, too, such as cherry, lemon, or coconut.

24 ounces vanilla Greek yogurt

2 teaspoons sugar

4 shots hot espresso or ¾ cup (6 ounces) strong brewed coffee

4 tablespoons chopped unsalted pistachios

4 tablespoons dark chocolate chips or shavings

Per Serving Calories: 270; Total Fat: 10g; Saturated Fat: 4g; Cholesterol: 9mg; Sodium: 119mg; Total Carbohydrates: 37g; Fiber: 2g; Protein: 11g

1. Spoon the yogurt into four bowls or tall glasses.

2. Mix ½ teaspoon of sugar into each of the espresso shots (or all the sugar into the coffee).

3. Pour one shot of hot espresso or 1.5 ounces of coffee over each bowl of yogurt.

4. Top each bowl with 1 tablespoon of pistachios and 1 tablespoon of chocolate chips and serve.

Prep tip: Chill your bowls or glasses ahead of time in the freezer for an extra layer of frostiness to contrast with the hot espresso.

Grilled Stone Fruit with Whipped Ricotta

NUT-FREE, GLUTEN-FREE, EGG-FREE, VEGETARIAN, 5 INGREDIENTS

An outdoor grill or a stove-top grill pan can quickly turn summer stone fruit, like peaches, nectarines, apricots, and plums, into caramelized sweet treats. Use ripe but firm fruit. Serena just recently discovered how light and fluffy whipped ricotta can be—it's her new go-to dessert topper.

Nonstick cooking spray

4 peaches or nectarines (or 8 apricots or plums), halved and pitted

2 teaspoons extra-virgin olive oil

¾ cup whole-milk ricotta cheese

1 tablespoon honey

¼ teaspoon freshly grated nutmeg

4 sprigs mint, for garnish (optional)

Per Serving Calories: 176; Total Fat: 9g; Saturated Fat: 4g; Cholesterol: 24mg; Sodium: 40mg; Total Carbohydrates: 20g; Fiber: 2g; Protein: 7g

1. Spray the cold grill or a grill pan with nonstick cooking spray. Heat the grill or grill pan to medium heat.

2. Place a large, empty bowl in the refrigerator to chill.

3. Brush the fruit all over with the oil. Place the fruit cut-side down on the grill or pan and cook for 3 to 5 minutes, or until grill marks appear. (If you're using a grill pan, cook in two batches.) Using tongs, turn the fruit over. Cover the grill (or the grill pan with aluminum foil) and cook for 4 to 6 minutes, until the fruit is easily pierced with a sharp knife. Set aside to cool.

4. Remove the bowl from the refrigerator and add the ricotta. Using an electric beater, beat the ricotta on high for 2 minutes. Add the honey and nutmeg and beat for 1 more minute. Divide the warm (or room temperature) fruit among 4 serving bowls, top with the ricotta mixture, and a sprig of mint (if using) and serve.

Ingredient tip: We love the super freshness and ease of grating nutmeg pods with a Microplane or citrus zester vs. using (less-fresh) jarred ground nutmeg. Fresh nutmeg pods are about the size of a small peach pit and are sold in the supermarket spice aisle.

Pomegranate-Quinoa Dark Chocolate Bark

DAIRY-FREE, NUT-FREE, GLUTEN-FREE, EGG-FREE, VEGETARIAN, 5 INGREDIENTS

This four-ingredient chocolate lover's treat is so easy to make and so yummy to eat, you may be inclined to whip up a batch weekly. We've paired dark chocolate with fruity, tart pomegranate seeds and nutty quinoa, which gives a burst of sweet and salt and a satisfying crunch factor. Deanna likes to make this bark around the holidays to give as a homemade gift (while making an extra batch for herself).

SERVES

6

PREP TIME

10

COOK TIME

5

CHILL TIME

10

Nonstick cooking spray

½ cup uncooked tricolor or regular quinoa

½ teaspoon kosher or sea salt

8 ounces dark chocolate or 1 cup dark chocolate chips

½ cup fresh pomegranate seeds

1. In a medium saucepan coated with nonstick cooking spray over medium heat, toast the uncooked quinoa for 2 to 3 minutes, stirring frequently. Do not let the quinoa burn. Remove the pan from the stove, and mix in the salt. Set aside 2 tablespoons of the toasted quinoa to use for the topping.

2. Break the chocolate into large pieces, and put it in a gallon-size zip-top plastic bag. Using a metal ladle or a meat pounder, pound the chocolate until broken into smaller pieces. (If using chocolate chips, you can skip this step.) Dump the chocolate out of the bag into a medium, microwave-safe bowl and heat for 1 minute on high in the microwave. Stir until the chocolate is completely melted. Mix the toasted quinoa (except the topping you set aside) into the melted chocolate.

CONTINUES NEXT PAGE

3. Line a large, rimmed baking sheet with parchment paper. Pour the chocolate mixture onto the sheet and spread it evenly until the entire pan is covered. Sprinkle the remaining 2 tablespoons of quinoa and the pomegranate seeds on top. Using a spatula or the back of a spoon, press the quinoa and the pomegranate seeds into the chocolate.

4. Freeze the mixture for 10 to 15 minutes, or until set. Remove the bark from the freezer, and break it into about 2-inch jagged pieces. Store in a sealed container or zip-top plastic bag in the refrigerator until ready to serve.

Ingredient tip: Experiment with using a few different colored quinoas, like white, red, and black, to provide a pretty color contrast on the chocolate bark.

Per Serving Calories: 283; Total Fat: 16g; Saturated Fat: 7g; Cholesterol: 2mg; Sodium: 169mg; Total Carbohydrates: 32g; Fiber: 5g; Protein: 4g

Lemon Fool

NUT-FREE, GLUTEN-FREE, EGG-FREE, VEGETARIAN, 5 INGREDIENTS

SERVES

4

PREP TIME

10

CHILL TIME

15

COOK TIME

5

You may think it's "foolish" to talk about a chilled dessert you can make in just 30 minutes. But our trick is to chill the mixing bowls, which helps reduce the amount of chill time. And if you've never made homemade whipped cream before, you'll be pleasantly surprised at how easy and amazing it is.

1 cup 2% plain Greek yogurt

1 medium lemon

¼ cup cold water

1½ teaspoons cornstarch

3½ tablespoons honey, divided

2/3 cup heavy (whipping) cream

Fresh fruit and mint leaves, for serving (optional)

1. Place a large glass bowl and the metal beaters from your electric mixer in the refrigerator to chill. Add the yogurt to a medium glass bowl, and place that bowl in the refrigerator to chill as well.

2. Using a Microplane or citrus zester, zest the lemon into a medium, microwave-safe bowl. Halve the lemon, and squeeze 1 tablespoon of lemon juice into the bowl. Add the water and cornstarch, and stir well. Whisk in 3 tablespoons of honey. Microwave the lemon mixture on high for 1 minute; stir and microwave for an additional 10 to 30 seconds, until the mixture is thick and bubbling.

3. Remove the bowl of yogurt from the refrigerator, and whisk in the warm lemon mixture. Place the yogurt back in the refrigerator.

CONTINUES NEXT PAGE

4. Remove the large chilled bowl and the beaters from the refrigerator. Assemble your electric mixer with the chilled beaters. Pour the cream into the chilled bowl, and beat until soft peaks form—1 to 3 minutes, depending on the freshness of your cream.

5. Take the chilled yogurt mixture out of the refrigerator. Gently fold it into the whipped cream using a rubber scraper; lift and turn the mixture to prevent the cream from deflating. Chill until serving, at least 15 minutes but no longer than 1 hour.

6. To serve, spoon the lemon fool into four glasses or dessert dishes and drizzle with the remaining ½ tablespoon of honey. Top with fresh fruit and mint, if desired.

Prep tip: After washing and drying lemons, oranges, or limes, zest the citrus rind directly into your bowl instead of onto a cutting board, where some of the flavorful oils will be left behind. Then roll the fruit on the counter, pressing firmly with your hand to break the juice sacs inside to release more of the liquid when juicing.

Per Serving Calories: 241; Total Fat: 16g; Saturated Fat: 10g; Cholesterol: 59mg; Sodium: 41mg; Total Carbohydrates: 21g; Fiber: 1g; Protein: 7g

Roasted Orange Rice Pudding

NUT-FREE, GLUTEN-FREE, VEGETARIAN

SERVES 6

PREP TIME 10

COOK TIME 20

Inspired by classic Italian caramelized oranges, these super sweet roasted orange slices are the crowning glory in this dreamy, creamy rice pudding, which can be served for dessert or breakfast. You can also use them to top yogurt, ice cream, cereal, or green salads.

Nonstick cooking spray

2 medium oranges

2 teaspoons extra-virgin olive oil

1/8 teaspoon kosher or sea salt

2 large eggs, beaten

2 cups 2% milk

1 cup 100% orange juice

1 cup uncooked instant brown rice

1/4 cup honey

1/2 teaspoon ground cinnamon

1 teaspoon vanilla extract

1. Preheat the oven to 450°F. Spray a large, rimmed baking sheet with nonstick cooking spray. Set aside.

2. Slice the unpeeled oranges into 1/4-inch rounds. Brush with oil, and sprinkle with salt. Place the slices on the baking sheet and roast for 4 minutes. Flip the slices and roast for 4 more minutes, until they begin to brown. Remove from the oven and set aside.

3. Crack the eggs into a medium bowl near the stove. In a medium saucepan, mix together the milk, orange juice, rice, honey, and cinnamon. Bring to a boil over medium-high heat, stirring constantly. Reduce the heat to medium-low and simmer for 10 minutes, stirring occasionally.

CONTINUES NEXT PAGE

4. Using a measuring cup, scoop out ½ cup of the hot rice mixture and whisk it into the eggs. Then, while constantly stirring the mixture in the pan, slowly pour the egg mixture back into the saucepan (to prevent the eggs from scrambling). Cook on low heat for 1 to 2 minutes, until thickened, stirring constantly; do not boil. Remove from the heat and stir in the vanilla.

5. Let the pudding stand for a few minutes for the rice to soften. The rice will be cooked but slightly chewy. For softer rice, let stand for another half hour. Serve warm or at room temperature, topped with the roasted oranges.

Ingredient tip: If your honey becomes hard and crystallized, it's still good to use. To liquefy crystallized honey, microwave 2 inches of water in a small, microwave-safe bowl for 30 seconds to 1 minute, until hot. Set the honey bottle in the water for a few minutes, until the honey is liquid again.

Per Serving Calories: 225; Total Fat: 6g; Saturated Fat: 2g; Cholesterol: 69mg; Sodium: 103mg; Total Carbohydrates: 39g; Fiber: 2g; Protein: 6g

Honey-Cherry Walnut Brownies

VEGETARIAN, ONE POT

SERVES
9

PREP
TIME
10

COOK
TIME
20

We're closing out our cookbook with the beloved American chocolate treat made a bit better for you with our Mediterranean pantry. We've cut back on the typical amount of sugar in most brownie recipes and swapped in some honey for an earthy and floral flavor. Walnuts and olive oil help boost the heart-healthy fat levels, and cherries give a surprise burst of color and juice in the middle of each brownie.

Nonstick cooking spray

½ cup sugar

⅓ cup honey

¼ cup extra-virgin olive oil

2 large eggs

1 teaspoon vanilla extract

½ cup 2% plain Greek yogurt

½ cup whole-wheat pastry flour

⅓ cup unsweetened dark chocolate cocoa powder

¼ teaspoon baking powder

¼ teaspoon salt

⅓ cup chopped walnuts

9 fresh cherries, stemmed and pitted, or 9 frozen cherries

Per Serving Calories: 225; Total Fat: 11g; Saturated Fat: 2g; Cholesterol: 42mg; Sodium: 89mg; Total Carbohydrates: 31g; Fiber: 1g; Protein: 5g

1. Preheat the oven to 375°F, and set the rack in the middle of the oven. Coat a 9-inch square baking pan with nonstick cooking spray.

2. In a stand mixer bowl or large bowl, beat the sugar, honey, and oil until well blended. Beat in the eggs and vanilla. Beat in the yogurt until the batter is smooth.

3. In a medium bowl, whisk together the flour, cocoa powder, baking powder, and salt. Add the flour mixture to the egg mixture and beat until all the dry ingredients are incorporated. Mix in the walnuts.

4. Pour the batter into the prepared pan. Push the cherries into the batter, three to a row in three rows, so one will be at the center of each brownie once you cut them into squares.

5. Bake the brownies for 18 to 20 minutes or until just set. Remove from the oven and place on a rack to cool for 5 minutes or so. Cut into nine squares and serve.

Ingredient tip: Switch up the fruit or nuts to your liking. Try blueberries with pecans or raspberries with almonds. And you can always omit the nuts for those with nut allergies.

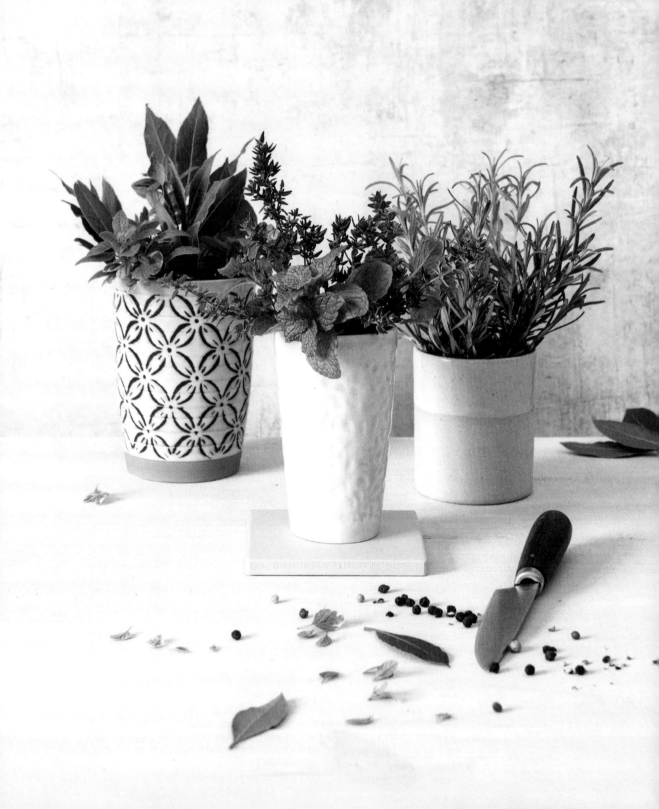

Conversion Tables

VOLUME EQUIVALENTS (LIQUID)

US Standard	US Standard (ounces)	Metric (approximate)
2 tablespoons	1 fl. oz.	30 mL
¼ cup	2 fl. oz.	60 mL
½ cup	4 fl. oz.	120 mL
1 cup	8 fl. oz.	240 mL
1½ cups	12 fl. oz.	355 mL
2 cups or 1 pint	16 fl. oz.	475 mL
4 cups or 1 quart	32 fl. oz.	1 L
1 gallon	128 fl. oz.	4 L

OVEN TEMPERATURES

Fahrenheit (F)	Celsius (C) (approximate)
250°F	120°C
300°F	150°C
325°F	165°C
350°F	180°C
375°F	190°C
400°F	200°C
425°F	220°C
450°F	230°C

VOLUME EQUIVALENTS (DRY)

US Standard	Metric (approximate)
1/8 teaspoon	0.5 mL
¼ teaspoon	1 mL
½ teaspoon	2 mL
¾ teaspoon	4 mL
1 teaspoon	5 mL
1 tablespoon	15 mL
¼ cup	59 mL
1/3 cup	79 mL
½ cup	118 mL
2/3 cup	156 mL
¾ cup	177 mL
1 cup	235 mL
2 cups or 1 pint	475 mL
3 cups	700 mL
4 cups or 1 quart	1 L

WEIGHT EQUIVALENTS

US Standard	Metric (approximate)
½ ounce	15 g
1 ounce	30 g
2 ounces	60 g
4 ounces	115 g
8 ounces	225 g
12 ounces	340 g
16 ounces or 1 pound	455 g

References

Ajala, O., et al. "Systematic Review and Meta-Analysis of Different Dietary Approaches to the Management of Type 2 Diabetes." *American Journal of Clinical Nutrition* 97, no. 3 (March 2013): 505–516 doi:10.3945/ajcn.112.042457.

Altomare, R., et al. "The Mediterranean Diet: A History of Health." *Iranian Journal of Public Health* 42, no. 5 (2013): 449–45.

Barak, Y., et al. "Impact of Mediterranean Diet on Cancer." *Cancer Genomics and Proteomics* 14, no. 66 (November/December 2017): 403–408 doi: 10.21873/cgp.20050.

Billingsley, H. E., et al. "The Antioxidant Potential of the Mediterranean Diet in Patients at High Cardiovascular Risk: An In-Depth Review of the PREDIMED." *Nutrition & Diabetes* 8, no. 1 (2018): 13 doi:10.1038/s41387-018-0025-1.

Hibbeln, J. R., J. M. Davis, C. Steer, P. Emmett, I. Rogers, C. Williams, and J. Golding. "Maternal Seafood Consumption in Pregnancy and Neurodevelopmental Outcomes in Childhood (ALSPAC Study): An Observational Cohort Study." *The Lancet* 369, no. 9561 (2007): 578–855 doi:10.1016/S0140-6736(07)60277-3.

International Pasta Organisation. *The Truth About Pasta*. Boston: Oldways Preservation Trust, 2016. Accessed June 15, 2018. https://oldwayspt.org/system/files/atoms/files/TruthAboutPasta16.pdf.

Luciano, M., et al. "Mediterranean-Type Diet and Brain Structural Change from 73 to 76 Years in a Scottish Cohort." *Neurology* 88, no. 5 (January 31, 2017): 229–455 doi:10.1212/WNL.0000000000003559.

Mozaffarian, D., and E. B. Rimm. "Fish Intake, Contaminants, and Human Health: Evaluating the Risks and the Benefits." *Journal of the American Medical Association* 296, no. 15 (November 2006):1885–1899 doi:10.1001/jama.296.15.1885.

Musumeci, G., F. M. Trovato, K. Pichler, A. M. Weinberg, C. Loreto, and P. Castrogiovanni. "Extra-Virgin Olive Oil Diet and Mild Physical Activity Prevent Cartilage Degeneration in an Osteoarthritis Model: An In Vivo and In Vitro Study on Lubricin Expression." *Journal of Nutritional Biochemistry* 24, no. 12 (December 2013): 2064–2075.

Oldways. "Oldways Mediterranean Diet Pyramid." Accessed June 20, 2018. https://oldwayspt.org/resources/oldways-mediterranean-diet-pyramid.

Pan, A., et al. "Red Meat Consumption and Mortality: Results from 2 Prospective Cohort Studies." *Archives of Internal Medicine* 172, no. 7 (2012): 555–563 doi:10.1001/archinternmed.2011.2287.

Papamichael, M. M., et al. "Does Adherence to the Mediterranean Dietary Pattern Reduce Asthma Symptoms in Children?" *Public Health Nutrition* 20, no. 15 (October 2017): 2722–2734 doi:10.1017/S1368980017001823.

Tan, Z. S., et al. "Red Blood Cell Omega-3 Fatty Acid Levels and Markers of Accelerated Brain Aging." *Neurology* 78, no. 9 (February 28, 2012): 658–664 doi:10.1212/WNL.0b013e318249f6a9.

U.S. Department of Agriculture. *Choose My Plate.* Accessed June 28, 2018. https://www.choosemyplate.gov/

U.S. Department of Health and Human Services and U.S. Department of Agriculture. *Dietary Guidelines for Americans 2015–2020*, 8th Edition. December 2015. Accessed June 15, 2018. https://health.gov/dietaryguidelines/2015/guidelines/.

U.S. News & World Report. "Best Diets Overall." January 3, 2018. https://health.usnews.com/best-diet/best-diets-overall.

Recipe Index

Index

Acknowledgments

We wouldn't be here today without the many food-loving dietitian colleagues and cherished friends we've met along the way, including Regan Jones, Robin Plotkin, Gretchen Brown, and Janice Bissex, who we've been lucky enough to collaborate with and celebrate with over the years during this crazy, delicious journey.

To one of the original spice girls, fearless entrepreneur, favorite roomie, and dear friend, Bonnie Johnson.

Shout out to all our family, friends, and neighbors, including Kate Thoelke, Dawn Schnare, Ellen Cohen, Donna Millius, and Catherine and Doug Stuart, who willingly taste-tested our dishes and provided honest feedback along the way.

Thank you to dietitian cookbook gurus, Marlene Koch, Ellie Krieger, Sally Kuzemchak, and Jackie Newgent for their mentoring and culinary nutrition inspiration.

To Rachel Tetlie, our enthusiastic intern, who was patient with us as we navigated our way through the writing process as new cookbook authors.

And a huge thank you to the entire Callisto Media editorial and design team, from Elizabeth Castoria, who championed our talent from the start; to Katie Moore, who held our hand every step of the way; all the way to Ann Edwards, who was invaluable in helping us launch our project into the world.

And lastly, much love and gratitude to our *Teaspoon of Spice* readers and followers who inspire us every day to keep seasoning everything with a little bit of nutrition and a whole lot of yum while still keeping things real.

About the Authors

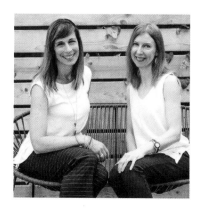

Serena Ball, MS, RDN, and Deanna Segrave-Daly, RDN, co-own Teaspoon Communications, LLC, and blog at TeaspoonOfSpice.com, where their motto is "Two dietitians who love food as much as you do." Both of them have over 20 years of food, nutrition, and culinary communications experience, and they've dedicated their careers to helping people get delicious and nutritious meals on the table. Most recently, Serena and Deanna have built up a dedicated readership and following by sharing their Healthy Kitchen Hacks and yummy, family-friendly recipes through their social media platforms and regular cooking segments on local TV stations. This is their first cookbook.

Serena lives in the country outside St. Louis, where she cooks in her bright, aqua-colored kitchen for her husband and four children, ages 5 to 13 years.

Deanna lives in suburban Philadelphia with her 11-year-old pizza-loving daughter, tricky-eater husband, and rescue cat.